'The topic of social injustice and its potential exacerbation and amplification in relation to the climate crisis is an important topic for art therapists to consider. Dr Bird suggests that the twin concepts of reflexivity and intersectionality are of crucial importance at this pivotal time. Bird notes a strand of art therapy which produces reductive narratives of deviancy and normality embedded in an atomised Capitalism which fails to properly acknowledge the communal and social aspects of experience, including environment. This book challenges our own ethics and practice. It challenges us, as a body of practitioners, to think about where we stand on the big issues of the day. I recommend it.'

Dr Susan Hogan, *PhD, D.Litt, is a Professor of Arts and Health at the University of Derby, College of Arts, Humanities and Education. Professorial Fellow, Institute of Mental Health, Nottingham.*

'Social action art therapy in times of crisis places the work of art therapy within an ecological and environmental context. The approaches described supports the reader to critically engage with the way that we think about the crisis we are living in and places the arts therapies within a socially engaged paradigm. The book shows how the use of art-based research and art therapy practice can contribute to making emotional sense of the climate crisis.'

Gary Nash, *Dip AT, MAAT, is a HCPC registered art therapist. Gary co-founded the London Art Therapy Centre in 2009, where he is a practitioner-researcher. He is a visiting lecturer at the Institute for Arts in Therapy and Education and the University of Hertfordshire. He is co-editor of* Environmental Arts Therapy, *Routledge, 2020.*

Social Action Art Therapy in a Time of Crisis

Social Action Art Therapy in a Time of Crisis outlines theories and models of social action art therapy, identifies its application in times of crisis, and explores the ways in which art therapy can work effectively for individuals and groups experiencing crisis.

Drawing upon various ecologies, climate psychology, and eco-art therapy, this book addresses various responses to climate change, including notions of belonging, the physicality of experience, and the role of imagination in creating alternative versions of the future. The author presents a social action approach to art therapy as a way of addressing the political and collective components of climate change as well as the individual and emotional components. To help explore what social action art therapy can offer in this time of crisis, the author illustrates examples that show how the ideas have been used in other moments of crisis, including asylum, refuge, and domestic abuse.

This innovative book contributes to the development of contemporary art therapy practice and will be of interest to arts therapists, arts psychotherapists, expressive therapists, ecotherapists, ecopsychologists, arts-based researchers, and many more.

Dr Jamie Bird is a senior lecturer and researcher based at the University of Derby, United Kingdom. He is an associate editor of the *International Journal of Art Therapy*.

Social Action Art Therapy in a Time of Crisis

Jamie Bird

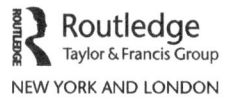
Routledge
Taylor & Francis Group

NEW YORK AND LONDON

Cover image: Magnolia 1 (Mixed media by Lor Bird)

First published 2023
by Routledge
605 Third Avenue, New York, NY 10158

and by Routledge
4 Park Square, Milton Park, Abingdon, Oxon, OX14 4RN

Routledge is an imprint of the Taylor & Francis Group, an informa business

© 2023 Jamie Bird

Library of Congress Cataloging-in-Publication Data
A catalog record for this title has been requested

ISBN: 978-0-367-69622-1 (hbk)
ISBN: 978-0-367-69621-4 (pbk)
ISBN: 978-1-003-14256-0 (ebk)

DOI: 10.4324/9781003142560

Typeset in Baskerville
by KnowledgeWorks Global Ltd.

In gratitude to my parents for loving me into being
In gratitude to Lor for being with me in love
In gratitude to the other-than-human for holding us all'

Contents

List of figures

Author biography

Dr Jamie Bird is an art therapist and arts-based researcher. He has been involved in the teaching of undergraduate, postgraduate, and doctoral students within the subjects of therapeutic arts and creative expressive therapies at the *University of Derby*, United Kingdom, since 2004. He has been an associate-editor of the *International Journal of Art Therapy* since 2018 and a board member of the *Climate Psychology Alliance* since 2021. He has an interest in the study of experiences through the use of creativity and imagination. He is also interested in generating quantitative data that measure the effectiveness of art therapy.

Preface

Jamie Bird

Setting out to write this book, at the end of the British summer of 2020, I embarked upon it like a pilgrimage. I had a desire to be guided as much by intuition, as much as I was by reason and cognitive analysis. Like a pilgrimage, it required faith and courage to set forth and to keep stepping forwards. Like a pilgrimage, it needed to be a journey with an intention. Unlike a pilgrimage, the exact location and essence of the destination would only be fully known and appreciated after the journey had come to an end, because the journey is one that needed to be open to new influences as the writing progressed. A journey that needed to be open to new characters met upon the road and of being led down unexpected pathways. Pilgrimages tend to be taken in the company of others, rather than being solitary ventures. Here, my main companions were those authors and thinkers who have lent me their thoughts and ideas, and those people who have taken part in the arts-based activities that I make reference to. The process of writing is one that embodies the message of the book, which is that the arts offer a way of being present in the world at this time and that there is a particular approach to art therapy that is able to address the needs of this time. That approach is social action art therapy, and the time is one of crisis and uncertainty.

The first and primary inspiration for setting out to write this book was my own growing sense of awareness about the reality of climate change. Scientific consensus shows that climate change is happening, is caused and exacerbated by human activity, and is now having a major and serious impact on all life on the Earth. The precise pace and location of those changes as they will appear in the future is part of an ongoing dialogue that has, on the one hand, proponents who argue that social collapse is inevitable within several decades (Bendell, 2018) and, on the other hand, those who argue that the evidence for such a collapse is not so clear (Nicholas et al., 2020). And as will be acknowledged repeatedly throughout this book, how that collapse plays out is contingent upon existing social hierarchies and injustices. Having gone through a process of emotional shock and grief, I arrived at the point where I was able to see that a valid response to that awareness, and the feelings that went with it, was to make use of what knowledge and skills I had at my disposal in order to assist others as they also came to terms with climate change. The grief and sadness was overwhelming at points, and it is still possible for me to be overwhelmed be the awareness that climate change brings. It is all too easy to move away from that awareness, whether intentionally or not, as a way of coping. But that turning away can only continue for so long before the feelings return. I am now a little better able to stay with those feelings, to welcome them as a valid empathic response to suffering, and to use those feelings to direct my actions in an intuitive way.

It is vitally important to state very clearly early on where my limitations are, and what I am not representing. I am not a climate or environmental scientist. I have tried my best to acquaint myself of such science and to keep abreast of it. The UN *Intergovernmental Panel on Climate Change* is a useful place to start for those who want to familiarise themselves with the most current scientific consensus about climate change. And whilst I have a good enough understanding of philosophy, sociology, and psychology, my primary area of knowledge is art therapy and it is other art therapists that this book is primarily written for.

When starting to write this book, the Covid-19 pandemic was continuing to spread globally, and the promise of a vaccine had yet to be fulfilled. As the writing comes to a close, it seems like only some progress has been made, with the unequal distribution of the vaccine globally revealing unequal relations between nations that were already there. We will likely be living with the restrictions that have been enacted by governments for a number of years to come and the longer-term implications of living with Covid-19 will continue to evolve. What is evident right now though is that the world has changed; or rather, many people have been changed by Covid-19. If I start with myself, I have been forced to be still and settled in one place, and I have made connections to other people and other ideas that might otherwise have passed me by. Those people and ideas were there at my margins already, but now they have become more central, and the way that their words resonate with me have become stronger. There has been the appearance of a pilgrimage taking place here also, where the journey has been an internal one, and where the final destination has not been some far-off exotic location, but one that is close by, in the present moment. Paying attention to what is in the immediate locality and moment in time has been powerful. A sense of being paused on the precipice.

At the same time as the appearance of a pandemic, there has been a resurgence of the *Black Lives Matter* movement, following the brutal, yet tragically ordinary and nonchalant, killing of George Floyd in the United States. This has led to an urgent sense of needing to better grasp the history of racism and colonialism, which in the United Kingdom has been woefully lacking in the individual consciousness of most white people – myself included – and the collective national narrative as propagated through the educational curriculum and through popular culture (Hirsch, 2018). Benefitting from a range of privileges that come from being a heterosexual white man, living and working within the United Kingdom, I have been challenged to uncover my own feelings of entitlement and sense of white supremacy and racism. This includes how I have been educated within a culture and nation that has chosen to simplify and obscure the historical relationship between itself and other cultures and nations. This has not been an easy process, which is as it should be. But I have been aided by others who have been willing to be allies and accomplices (the *Radical Therapist Network*[2] and the *Climate Psychology Alliance* in particular[3]), as we respond together to what this time is calling us to attend to. I have been helped in my engagement with this process through being able to recall the experience of gaining a better understanding of gender-based violence as a male researcher (Bird, 2019). An important element of that understanding has been an appreciation of how the twin concepts of reflexivity and intersectionality can enable an appreciation of both divergence and similarity between people in a considered way. Within United Kingdom art therapy practice, addressing white privilege and anti-racist work is now more explicitly addressed (Eastwood, 2021).

At the start of this pilgrimage then, my acceptance of the climate crisis was already present. Covid-19 and the *Black Lives Matter* movement further revealed the reality of our vulnerability and interconnectedness as a whole species of *Homo sapiens* as well as highlighting how racism distorts that interconnection and vulnerability, so that some peoples are safer than others. And how do we even maintain an idea of what being human means when we comprehend that there are roughly as many other-than-human cells within the human body as there are exclusively human cells? Or that our DNA retains traces of so many other species (Margulis and Sagan, 1987). It is this sort of knowledge that leads to a reframing of the boundaries between the human and other-than-human, and which disrupts ordinary ideas of ancestry and heritage, and which has increasingly come to define how I consider my own sense of being human.

In considering my response, as an art therapist and researcher, to the various crises we face, I am taken with the words of Timothy Morton: 'It is very much the job of philosophers and other humanities scholars to attune ourselves to the upgrading process and to help explain it' (2013, p. 101). The upgrading process that Morton refers to is the shift in human awareness and being that global warming entails. Art therapy is aligned strongly with the humanities in the way that it places creativity and imagination, as both a means and an end, at the core of how it thinks about and responds to the human condition. The sort of upgrading that Morton suggests is now required is one that opens up the very meaning of the concepts of 'human,' 'nature,' and 'world.' Such a fundamental shift needs more than a cognitive level of analysis and understanding. Intuition, imagination, ancient, and sacred knowledge will have to be called upon as much as rationality and empiricism as we leave the benign-for-humans climate of the Holocene behind and enter a new realm where the straight edges of modernity and the perpetual search for profit, material growth, and convenience can no longer guide us.

This book then brings together my experience of synthesising social action art therapy, arts-based research methods, and participatory research methods to show how art therapy can offer an effective way to work with individuals and groups who have encountered times of crisis in their lives. It focuses on three specific sets of experiences of crisis: asylum and refuge, domestic violence and abuse, and climate change. I argue that those moments and times of crisis are similar in terms of how they can be framed as expressions of particular features of modernity – the use of state-sanctioned violence to maintain hierarchies of power and control, and the valuing of human rationality above all other ways of knowing and being – and how they share certain salient features. Those features include transitions between places and ways of being as a consequence of crisis, the remaking of a sense of belonging and self post-crisis, and the importance of place and objects within the creation and sustainment of that renewed sense of belonging. This last feature is of relevance where crisis disrupts both the physical and relational qualities of belonging. This includes the loss of home, loss of landscape, loss of family, and a mourning for the real and for the imagined.

I argue that for art therapy to engage with the sorts of crisis identified, it has to take account of the social and political contexts within which these crises emerge and that art therapists operate within. It is hoped that this book will be able to sit alongside those existing and forthcoming publications that aim to assist art therapists to work in this time of crisis, that it helps with the process of transition and adaptation required, and that it might be a welcome companion on someone else's pilgrimage.

Notes

1 https://www.ipcc.ch/ [accessed: 5/1/2022]
2 https://www.radicaltherapistnetwork.com/ [accessed: 5/1/2022]
3 https://www.climatepsychologyalliance.org/ [accessed: 5/1/2022]

References

Bendell, J. 2018. *Deep Adaptation: A Map for Navigating Climate Tragedy*. IFLAS Occasional Paper 2, https://www.lifeworth.com/deepadaptation.pdf (accessed 23/6/22).

Bird, J. 2019. "The Eye of the Beholder": Encountering women's Experience of Domestic Violence and Abuse as a Male Researcher and Art Therapist. *In:* HOGAN, S. (ed.) *Arts Therapies and Gender Issues: International Perspectives on Research*. London: Routledge.

Eastwood, C. 2021. White privilege and art therapy in the UK: are we doing the work? *International Journal of Art Therapy*, 26, 1–9.

Hirsch, A. 2018. *Brit(Ish): On Race, Identity and Belonging*. London: Vintage.

Margulis, L. & Sagan, D. 1987. *Microcosmos: Four Billion Years of Evolution from Our Microbial Ancestors*. New York: Summit.

Morton, T. 2013. *Hyperobjects: Philosophy and Ecology after the End of the World*. Minnesota: University of Minessota Press.

Nicholas, T., Hall, G. & Schmidt, C. 2020. *The faulty science, doomism, and flawed conclusions of Deep Adaptation*. Open Democracy [Online]. Available: https://www.opendemocracy.net/en/oureconomy/faulty-science-doomism-and-flawed-conclusions-deep-adaptation/ [Accessed 1/10/2021].

Acknowledgements

This book is the product of many years of work, developing ideas, and ways of working. During that slow process of development, I have been supported, inspired, and educated by many people: teachers, supervisors, peers, colleagues, and students. In no particular order, this includes Judie Taylor, Ursula Newell-Walker, Susan Hogan, Maggie O'Neill, Cath Wakeman, Becky Barnes, Linda Wheildon, Sage Stephanou, Mandy Rowland-Smith, Dena Trossell, Connie Friedrich, and Val Huet. Many of these relationships are a consequence of my long connection to the *University of Derby*, United Kingdom, and I am grateful for the opportunities that institution has provided me with. A special thanks goes to all those allies in the *Climate Psychology Alliance* and the *Radical Therapist Network* for providing a valuable space to think, feel, and dream during these beautifully weird times. Finally, heartfelt gratitude to Lor Bird for her unwavering belief in me and for the gift of her creativity.

1 Introduction

This first chapter sets out the historical and political context within which the ideas I explore in subsequent chapters are placed. This is a very particular moment in time, in which climate change has an increasing impact upon all aspects of personal, social, and political life; a time in which a global-scale phenomena, generations in the making, is increasingly having an impact upon all aspects of our lives as humans, and all aspects of the other-than-human world. The scientific consensus is clear. Human action has increased the level of carbon dioxide and methane in the atmosphere, which in turn is having a significant causal impact upon average global temperatures and local weather patterns. At the same time, industrial activity has accelerated rates of extinction and biodiversity loss. Pollution is changing the fabric of water and soil. This book is primarily concerned with how art therapists can continue to work, when the knowledge of this crisis becomes urgent for them and for those people and groups they work with. Where knowledge of how the changing climate created by global warming causes emotional pain and disturbance, it can be difficult to hold on to ways of working that can often feel remote and not relevant to the urgency that it appears to demand. A fundamental feature of climate change is that it transcends so many of the boundaries and belief systems that have been constructed by many, though not all, human civilisations. This includes the boundaries of national borders, of time-frames, and of categories of being. A powerful way of conceptualising this comes in philosopher Timothy Morton's observation that global warming is a *hyperobject* (Morton, 2013). I will say more about this important feature of global warming, as it pertains to what I explore in this book, further on in this chapter. Fundamentally, it alludes to global warming being a species-level event that is spread across hundreds, if not thousands of years, in to the past and the future, and which is too large an event for any individual human to comprehend cognitively or to come to terms with emotionally, or to be at peace with spiritually. How do we, as humans, as art therapists, carry on, when the foundations of what we take for granted are being eroded and undermined? How do we make sense

DOI: 10.4324/9781003142560-1

of the science and the competing interpretations of how to respond to what science is predicting? What is an appropriate response to such a crisis that does not inadvertently repeat the causes of the crisis, and how might that response come from a place of reflection rather than reaction?

This book is for those art therapists who have some grasp of the magnitude of climate change. It is for those who are emotionally affected by climate change as art therapists and want to think about how they can stay with difficult truths and complex emotions so that they can continue working effectively as art therapists. It is for art therapists who are working with clients who are emotionally affected by climate change, and want some pointers and examples of how they can be of help to those clients. This is not a book about working with climate change sceptics, nor is it a primer on the science of climate change. And whilst there is the outlining of some basic climate science details, and some exploration of the emotional components of climate change scepticism, readers are directed to the plentiful supply of resources that address those particular topics in far greater detail. What this book aims to do is to introduce into art therapy discourse and practice a more thorough and nuanced understanding of ecological and environmental thought, within the context of climate crisis. This is not to discount what already exists around the practice of environmental art therapy (Heginworth, 2009; Heginworth and Nash, 2019) and nature-based expressive therapies (Atkins and Snyder, 2018), but rather to complement those practices by focusing in detail on the very particular features of climate crisis that are likely to be pertinent to art therapists now and over the coming decade. Within that focus, psychological and socio-political perspectives are given equal weight, and thus the adoption of a social action and social justice approach to art therapy.

A qualification about particular words that I frequently use in this book is required early on. The word crisis appears often. It is in the very title of the book. It frequently replaces the word 'change,' both here and in wider public discourse, when referring to climate change. Crisis, as a political term, has varied and complex meanings (Mcconnell, 2020). It occupies a similar role as the word 'emergency' in this context. Climate crisis and climate emergency are terms used by many activists, lobbyists, and authors because it communicates the magnitude of the problem better than the more passive and benign term climate change. Change suggests that we always have agency over what is happening. There is though a problem in referring to crisis and emergency. Crisis and emergency demands a response. It suggests that a solution must be found – and will be found – at all costs and as rapidly as possible, when a more measured and considered response might actually be a truly radical way of understanding what caused the crisis, and how we might resolve those causes. Careful attention also has to be paid to how the manufacturing of a feeling of crisis is a frequent method of social control, through the instigation of policies that curtail the freedoms of usually already vulnerable groups, in order to garner political votes through the appearance of being strong on law and order. For example, the fear of 'muggers' (code for young black men) in Britain (Hall et al., 1978), and the so-called super-predators (code for young black and Latino men) in the United States, was exploited and magnified by various political parties to appeal to certain groups of voters (most usually older white voters) during the 1970s and 1980s. A more contemporary and ongoing example is how those seeking refuge and political asylum in Europe are presented as being part of a migration crisis, even though the numbers arriving in 2020 are a fraction of their 2015[1] peak. A further reason for the terms crisis and emergency, in the context of climate and ecology, being potentially problematic, is that their use suggests that the ecological consequences of human activity is only now, in the early 20th century, being realised and challenged, therefore hiding the long history of dissent, warning voices and alternative visions of how modernity might have been developed. Modernity creates a perpetual state of crisis and revolution through its desire to reach and meet its twin goals of domination and emancipation (Latour, 1993). As such, it is important to be aware that the idea of states of crises is certainly not new, nor is the global scale of those crises. There is also the observation made by Jiddu Krishnamurti as to where any crisis is truly located: 'The crisis is not economic, war, the bomb, the politicians, the scientists, but the crisis is within us, the crisis is our consciousness' (Krishnamurti, 1992, p. 86). This is a vitally important distinction to take account of. It does not mean that we should not act, but that we take account of the thoughts that act as the foundations of action. It fits with the common reframe that the tools and methods of modernity are unfit to fix the problems of modernity; that the master's tools cannot dismantle the master's house (Lorde, 2018).

Transition is perhaps a better way of framing and approaching the topics addressed in this book. Crisis suggest a state of flux and rupture. It suggests one state coming to an end and another beginning, but in an uncontrolled or unpredictable way. That is a major challenge to any sense of being in control. Transition suggests a change between states that can be managed. Adaptation serves a similar role. Both evoke planning and preparation for future events. The concept of transition became a major part of my thinking about domestic abuse and it also has its place in thinking about migration and about climate change. The task then becomes one of turning times of crises into processes of transition.

Related to thinking critically about that use of the word crisis is the range of terms used to refer to the changes in climate and environment that this book is concerned with. Climate change is frequently used, but does not do full justice to what that change actually is. It is the term more often used when action is not deemed urgent or necessary. Global warming or global heating are more accurate in identifying that change and suggest more urgent responses. Likewise, when using the words 'world' or 'nature,' there is a need to preface this with a caution against oversimplification or the transposing of one notion of them onto others and to ask the questions: *whose 'world'; whose 'nature'?* Any reference to nature is fraught with problems, especially so where nature is represented as being in a state that is unspoilt, pristine, virgin, or wild. Such representations can fail to take account of the historical effects – both harmonious and destructive – of human inter-actions with land, water, and animals. The misconception about the size and diversity of societies in the Americas, and their shaping of nature before European contact in 1492, is a good example of such a failure (Mann, 2012).

The second group of terms that need critical consideration is the use of the pronouns 'we' and 'us,' and the collective nouns 'humans' and 'species.' Where they do appear, it can all too easily suggest a glob-ally homogenous community of people that share similar experiences of, and responsibilities for, climate change. Or, imply that they have equal access to the means of responding and adapting to it. This is not borne out by what is observed in the differences between countries, as they exist now and as they have existed in the past. In particular, the extraction of resources from the continents of Africa, the Americas, and Asia for use within the industrialising countries of Europe and North America from the 18th century onwards, and the later export-ing of polluting and exploitative industries in the opposite direction. The words 'us' and 'human' present similar challenges to the word 'we.' A presentation and understanding of global heating, and the idea of the anthropocene more broadly, that does not take account of history, risks flattening differences of responsibility between nations, and between groups of people within nations. Bonneuil and Fressoz write that the 'dominant narrative of the Anthropocene presents an abstract humanity uniformly involved – and, it implies, uniformly to blame' (2017, p. 66). Their argument being that both the humanities and Earth system sciences need to take full account of the historical flow of resources and power between different parts of the world and different elements of society. And if there is to be a broadening out of perspectives, indigenous ecological knowledge shows that there is a need to consider how the use of pro-nouns and collective nouns might preclude a consideration of other-than-human beings in thought and action (Kimmerer, 2020). Chapter 3, which includes an examination of modernity, will present a more nuanced examination of these arguments.

The anthropocene

The scientific features of climate change are outlined in this chapter but are not overly dwelt upon. Instead, climate change is explored from a sociological, psychological, and philosophical perspective. There is increasing acknowledgment that humans have had a significant detrimental impact upon the natural environment. Human activity has changed the normal cycles of global heating and cooling. The byproducts of agriculture and manufacturing have deposited huge quantities of chemicals and plastics into the soil, atmosphere, rivers, and oceans. A consequence of these human interactions is the accelerated extinction of species, a reduction in biodiversity, and the development of chaotic weather patterns. The *Intergovernmental Panel on Climate Change* (IPCC) stated in 2018 that 'Human activities are estimated to have caused approximately 1.0°C of global warming above pre-industrial levels [circa 1750], with a likely range of 0.8°C to 1.2°C. Global warming is likely to reach 1.5°C between 2030 and 2052 if it continues to increase at the current rate' (IPCC, 2018, p. 4) adding that there is a high level of confidence that this will occur if reduction in CO_2 emissions are not curtailed. This figure of an additional 1.5°C of warming by 2052 is viewed as an underestimate by those who draw attention to the conservative nature of IPCC reports (Spratt and Dunlop, 2018). Indeed the most recent IPCC report has revised the estimates upwards slightly (Masson-Delmotte et al., 2021). Best estimates indicate 1.6°C above pre-industrial levels occurring between 2041 and 2060 *if* emissions are drastically cut and net zero is reached by 2050. That estimate rises to 2.0°C if current emissions continue without reduction. Any acceleration of emissions, either through direct human activity, or the effects of melting ice sheets and the exposure of biomass, adds to that figure. If current rates of emissions rise only at the rate they have been over the last 30 years, the estimate is that the global average temperatures between 2080 and 2100 will be an additional 2.4°C to 4.2°C above today's average temperature[2]. To add to this is the theory of tipping points, whereby changes occur within a normally stable system that are both rapid and non-linear, so that a new state of stability is reached. The global average temperature that has sustained settled human societies over the last ten to twelve millennia, and can thus be considered a stable state, is coming to an end. What the new stable state will be, when it will be arrived at, and how favourable it will be to the continuation of human societies is unclear. But that change is coming, no matter what mitigating or adaptive changes are made in the short term. The time lag between emissions of carbon dioxide, methane and nitrogen oxide, fluorinated gases and their effect upon the global heating of the atmosphere and the oceans, and between global heating and events like glacial melting and the subsequent rise in sea levels, are far too slow to respond to rapid changes in emissions. These are process that are measured in centuries and millennia. It will likely take less time to make any attempt at addressing them or to learn to adapt to them, but those attempts stretch forward beyond most peoples' lifetimes. A key feature of the strangeness of global warming, that can make it so disorientating, is this stretching of time. When exactly is 'now' and what is short-term when the overall time scale is so other-than-human.

To take account of these long-term and non-reversible processes, a new geological term has been proposed to reflect the human-made element of this period in Earth's history: the anthropocene. The anthropocene, as a tentative geological term, appeared towards the turn of the 21st century (Crutzen, 2002). To begin with, the European industrial revolution, starting in the middle of the 18th century, was used as the marker for its beginning. Later definitions have placed that starting point as late 1945, with the first use of atomic weapons, and as early as the dawn of the Neolithic era, circa 8000 BCE, with the invention of agriculture, the domestication of animals, and the systematic use of deforestation. The anthropocene, as a concept, is a useful lens through which to view and think about climate change. In part, this is because it is a contested and problematic term which opens up ways of considering climate change from a range of perspectives. This includes views of climate change from the perspectives of Earth system sciences, economics and politics, sociology and anthropology, and humanities and philosophy. Bonneuil and Fressoz (2017) themselves suggest that other labels might better represent the complex interface between Earth sciences, history, and politics: the term 'capitalocene' for example reflects better how it is modern industrial manufacturing and agricultural processes, in the pursuit of ever expanding profits, which are the primary drivers of emissions and the erosion of air, soil, and water quality. The position I take is to approach the idea of the anthropocene from a perspective that takes account of the emotional components of the anthropocene, and the impact that comes from its unfolding influence.

To use one metaphor, the web and knot of natural connections that holds us as humans is coming apart. Coming apart in terms of the web of interconnections of climate, soil, and water, and in terms of the human constructions of material and immaterial objects. This includes values and beliefs about the relationship between the human and the other-than-human. It will change in ways, that as a species, we have not had to contend with before. Some projections point to a time when it will cease to sustain us. The benign climate that has served our agricultural and technological societies well for ten thousand years or so will becomes less stable. Crops will fail; fresh water will become scarce. Globally, many people have been sent down this road already due to imperialism, colonialism, extractive capitalism, and the environmental degradation that has been ongoing for generations. That road will get wider and wider as it sweeps up more and more people. This realisation is one part of what makes idea of the anthropocene so shocking (Bonneuil and Fressoz, 2017); the realisation that we have been living in the anthropocene for a long time – all the way back to the development of agriculture perhaps (Ruddiman, 2005; Lewis and Maslin, 2018) – and that social and environmental injustices are of one and the same source; namely hierarchy and the organisation of scarcity. The sense of shock also comes from the realisation that any awareness of the detrimental impact human choices have upon the environment is not a recent occurrence. Neither have those choices been accidental or unconscious. The anthropocene is a consequence of a consistent and wilful desire to exploit and manipulate Earth systems in order benefit human societies. The shock also comes from realising that none of this is accidental or the result of unconscious choices. It is too consistent, rational, and logical to be that. It was planned. In the same way that trans-Atlantic slavery was planned, the Holocaust was planned, the dropping of atomic bombs on Japan was planned. We can point to zones of ignorance that exist around human activity, but that is not the same as saying that those activities were, or are, a product of unconscious choice. Certainly not at a societal or collective level. In addition, just as the choice to exploit and deplete natural resources has been a feature of the history of many human societies, so too is there a parallel history of dissenting voices within those societies. Whilst those dissenting voices are now louder than they have ever been, they are not a new phenomenon. Traditional and indigenous ecological knowledge has shown great sensitivity to environmental change over many generations (Chisholm Hatfield et al., 2018). Neither are those voices that express an explicit denial of the detrimental impact of human choices upon the environment, or seek to distract or divert attention from attempts to address that impact, of recent origin.

In thinking about how scientists struggle to understand why a general acceptance of climate change has been slow to materialise, Bonneuil and Fressoz note that the anthropocene is shocking now in the same way that Charles Darwin's theory of evolution was shocking during the 19th century (2017). Many struggled to make sense of Darwin's ideas then, and a great proportion of people across the globe still reject the theory of natural selection and evolution for religious reasons. Arguably, the idea of the anthropocene presents as big a challenge to how the relationship between the human and the other-than-human is understood as the theory of evolution does.

Ecologies

Returning to the metaphor of the web, it is not a conscious rejection of a species from the world, but rather a species falling through the gaps in the web. And what might remain of the web of relationships between people, as the other-than-human web changes? This is the part that needs strengthening and nurturing. Work needs to be done to strengthen the bonds of connection and belonging between humans and between humans and the other-than-human. To do that work, there is a need, I would argue, to become ecological in both thought and action. And if there is a need to become more ecological, it is necessary to consider some of the different ways in which ecology has been conceptualised. So, I want to introduce three expressions of contemporary ecology thought that I think are worth considering in some detail. They are: deep ecology, developed by philosopher Arne Næss; dark ecology, as it appears within the writings of Timothy Morton; and social ecology, formulated and ardently defended by political activist and theorist Murray Bookchin. Each of those ecologies have their own distinct components, have clashed at points, but have enough features in common to hold them simultaneously in mind. In particular, each of them in their own way advocates the dissolving of a clear-cut boundary between the human and the other-than-human as a way of responding to ecological problems. Finally, in addition to these contemporary, and primarily western, ecologies, there is the much larger and older collection of indigenous and traditional ecological knowledge. An introduction to this traditional body of knowledge is provided, observing how traditional knowledge, meanings, and practices resonate with contemporary ecological thought.

Deep ecology

Starting with deep ecology, Arne Næss (1990) espoused a philosophy in which each person is encouraged to develop their own ecological philosophy (what Næss terms ecosophy) through constant critical questioning of ecological assumptions and through direct physical engagement with the natural world. The reference to depth within deep ecology comes from the challenge to constantly question ecological assumptions. Deep ecology applies a philosophical and psychological lens to understanding ecology and the relationship between the human and the other-than-human. This approach has sometimes been placed in contrast to the so-called shallow ecology, which is perceived to focus only on practical or political solutions to ecological problems; solutions such as sustainability, conservation, and preservation, which do not question the fundamental relationship between the human and the other-than-human. Applying the labels of deep and shallow to ecology have however fallen out of use due to the hierarchical overtone that their use implies. Warwick Fox (1995) instead proposes that transpersonal ecology is a more appropriate term to use in place of deep ecology. Reference to the transpersonal builds upon Næss' incorporation of the work of the 17th-century rationalist philosopher Baruch Spinoza (b1632, d1677) and that of political and spiritual leader Mahatma Gandhi (b1869, d1948) into his own philosophy. Spinoza blurs the distinction between God (specifically, the Judaic and Christian God) and nature, arguing that they are the totality of all, that they are one and the same substance, and therefore not able to be transcended through reason. For Spinoza, we cannot think ourselves outside of nature or of God. We instead come to know nature through our physical interaction with the physical world, and by implication we come to know god through our physical interaction with nature. This was heretical in the 17th-century Netherlands, and arguably just as antithetical to much of modernist philosophy, with its emphasis upon reason and logic, since that time. The element of Gandhi's teachings that Næss draws substantially from is Mahayana Buddhism, in particular the idea of bodhisattva, whereby self-actualisation and enlightenment are ongoing processes rather than static states of being. Bodhisattva is centred on developing compassion for all creation, and not being content until all suffering is overcome, as opposed to achieving enlightenment for oneself only. Deep ecology thus incorporates a spiritual understanding of the relationship between the human and the other-than-human; a position that reappears in many forms within contemporary ecological thought and practice.

In practical terms, deep ecology places particular emphasis upon the importance of maintaining, protecting, and expanding areas of natural wilderness. This emphasis upon wilderness within deep ecology finds its expression in historical and contemporary calls for re-wilding as a method of combating biodiversity loss, carbon sequestration, and flood mitigation. Another element of this desire for unspoilt, untamed, and wild places is the argument that greater familiarity with such places is both good for different aspects of being – physical, mental, and spiritual – and for encouraging a greater desire to protect and care for natural environments. The very contemporary expression of this line of thinking appears within the increasing body of evidence that supports the hypothesis that connecting with nature leads to enhanced levels of physical and mental wellbeing (Mcewan et al., 2021), and with greater levels of pro-environmental behaviour (Richardson et al., 2019). Ecotherapies of various types, including environmental art therapy and nature-based expressed therapy, echo this emphasis upon reconnection, and frequently incorporate spiritual practice and ritual into their own practice.

Critiques of deep ecology – particularly from a social ecology perspective (Bookchin, 1989) – are that there is the danger of the appearance of nihilism and misanthropy within its articulation of the effects of humans upon the land, and of adopting a depoliticised view of ecology, which risks being co-opted into eco-fascist rhetoric. For example, advocating for population control in the global south combined with fears of uncontrolled migration into the global north. It is also criticised for moving too quickly from being concerned about the environment to ideas of spiritual salvation along with the worship of nature-based gods and goddesses that are taken out of their cultural and historical contexts. From a social ecology perspective, such spirituality and worship slips too easily into irrational and wishful thinking, and to the formation of the kinds of power hierarchies that social ecology seeks to critique and overturn (Bookchin, 1989, Bookchin, 1993). Elsewhere, Morton (2013) argues that the nihilism that can creep into deep ecology has the potential to perpetuate an approach that is dualistic in its division between the human and the other-than-human, where human social spaces are framed as being un-natural and always in conflict with nature.

Dark ecology

In the form that philosopher Timothy Morton articulates it, dark ecology offers a playful and provocative version of ecology for the 21st century. A key example is how Morton argues that global warming and mass extinction are examples of what he terms hyperobjects (2013). Hyperobjects are those phenomena they are too large and too dispersed to take in as a single entity. They are too stretched and smeared across space and time for any one individual to comprehend. They resemble oncoming comets that slowly fill the sky rather than rush down towards us. They also, paradoxically, have the appearance of spectres that are barely observable in our peripheral vision. Arguably, in the short space of time since Morton first articulated those thoughts, the pressing reality of global warming means that its appearance is neither slow or at the periphery. And it never has been on the periphery for those many peoples who have been living with its consequences for many generations. Nevertheless, if global warming and mass extinction are to be classed as hyperobjects, then so also should the feelings that they provoke. The multitude of feelings that do arise – anxiety, grief, shock, guilt – are an indication of the scope and scale of these hyperobjects. A fundamental insight here is that climate crisis produces too many feelings for any single individual to hold alone. In the same way that no single individual is responsible for all of climate change – either its causes or its solutions – it takes collective effort to appreciate the reality of global warming and mass extinction, and to comprehend what they do to us emotionally as humans.

In another provocative turn, Morton refers to agrilogistics as a primary underlining cause of the predicament we collectively face as a species (Morton, 2016). By agrilogistics, Morton is referring to the invention of farming and urban living that appeared in various places between twelve and seven thousand years ago, practiced by the Palaeolithic and Chalcolithic people of the Fertile Crescent, the Yangtze river basin, and Mesoamerica. Agrilogistics is the formation of a way of thinking about the world that has acted, to repeat Morton's metaphor, as an operating system within which all religions and philosophies that have emerged during recorded history run like apps. Its key tenets are the separation of the human from the other-than-human, the formation of rigid social and political hierarchies, and the use of the mathematical process of addition, subtraction, multiplication, and division to manage the natural and human worlds. We cannot now easily re-write that operating system. Who we are, and the world we have created for ourselves, is entirely coded on top of that system. We have created a machine, in the form of settled and urbanised civilisations that now cannot be easily controlled or stopped. It is a fine example of a wicked problem, where any solution cannot be tested first, and the outcome of any actions taken now will not become clear for generations. A problem whose solutions require major sacrifices regardless of the direction taken. Given that all our religious, philosophical, and political structures are products of that agricultural mind-set, we cannot easily think outside of them. We would have to in some way recover, restore, or reinvent a nomadic hunter-gatherer mind-set, where the ownership of land and property by individuals is forsaken for the common good. The possibility – let alone the psychological or political desire – of doing that now in any kind of scaled-up systemic way, rapidly enough to make any difference to global heating over the coming century, are precisely zero (social ecology argues that the creation of common ownership of resources at a local level is more of a realistic possibility). What is more, human history, as Depesh Chakrabarty (2009) suggests, offers no guide to thinking or acting on a global scale about climate catastrophe. Whilst traditional ecological knowledge and indigenous people's responses to histories of social and ecological injustice offer an indication of what responses might look like at a communal or localised scale (Estes, 2019), no existing practices provide a total guide for the global-level change required. Global heating and mass extinction change what being human means, because the formalised ways of framing and managing the relationship between the human and the other-than-human – religion, philosophy, science – no longer work as expected. Some religions are able to imagine and work with entropy, extinction, and annihilation better than others – Buddhism for example – but most current systems of thought and belief do not provide the necessary philosophical tools to make sense of and thus respond appropriately to climate crisis.

Dark ecology has some thought-provoking things to say about time, of how we are required to hold in mind multiple versions of time simultaneously in order to make sense of climate crisis. Thinking ecologically – including thinking about global heating and mass extinction – means holding in mind different time scales simultaneously:

the moment-to-moment management of strong emotional reactions to experiences and reports of climate crisis; the way in which the seasons can be observed to be shifting in tone and character within a single lifetime; the global heating upon the melting of ice sheets measured in centuries and millennia. Morton observes that these differing time scales do not flow into each other seamlessly, as modernity would have us believe. Instead, they are granular and spikey. How can we, from the perspective of a single human lifespan, or even from within collective generational memory, comprehend what 100,000 years looks or feels like? Because that is one predicted long-term impact upon the rise of sea-levels as a consequence of anthropogenic heating, regardless of what we do now to mitigate our actions.

A critique of dark ecology is that it can appear to be too universalising in its reference to whole species events, and in terms of not fully taking account of the diversity of thought and relationship with the natural world across cultures and across history. It might also easily be co-opted by those who wish to do nothing or want to adopt a defeatist position, when there is an emphasis given to individuals not being responsible for climate change. However, a careful reading of Morton, and listening to him challenge the appearance of sexism and racism within academia and environmental organisations, reveals that such criticisms are ill-founded. And rather than being defeatist, Morton puts forward a call to be playful and artful in our response to the crisis that we face. Whilst no one can be individually held responsible for climate change, Morton proposes that we should separate responsibility from guilt. Once known, social and environmental injustice should be acted upon responsibly – or responded to in a just way – even if no single individual can be held accountable for their existence. Taken as a whole, dark ecology is primarily a psychological analysis of the meaning of climate crisis, and Morton's very personal account of his own emotional struggles and fears is helpful in showing how powerful these feelings are, but also how they have to be named and addressed collectively if they are not to become overwhelming.

Social ecology

If deep ecology and dark ecology point to philosophical and psychological understandings of the relationship between the other-than-human and the human, social ecology presents the hypothesis that the formation of social hierarchies are the foundation for both social and environmental injustices, positing that the two injustices are inseparable and 'that their resolution necessitates the most wide ranging social revolution possible as a means to avert ecological collapse' (Price, 2012, p. 159). All three ecologies share the idea that humans have, in most modern industrial societies, placed themselves above or outside the other-than-human. What social ecology adds to that understanding, as extensively developed by Murray Bookchin (Bookchin, 1989, Bookchin, 1993, Bookchin, 2015), is a nuanced examination of the hierarchical structures that create inequalities, exploitation, extraction, slavery, and colonialism, across and between class, gender, and race – starting first within human to human relationships before being extended out to human to other-than-human relationships. Phrases such as 'we are all in the same boat' that are used to communicate the global scale of the climate crisis come apart when one considers how some places are already a long way into living with climate catastrophe. We (the global and species-level we) might all be on the same ocean, but there are many kinds of boats on that ocean. Some of those boats are sinking; some have already sunk. The social mind-set that views people as a resource ripe for extraction is of the same mind-set that views land, plants, and animals as resources to be extracted and exploited. Social ecology makes explicit the links between colonialism and ecological breakdown and is therefore especially pertinent when considering the disparity between the global north and global south. If the 'shock of the anthropocene' is that we have been living inside a human-made climate for many centuries – for millennia even – and that the geological present can be extended far into the past and the future, the shock of the colonial (from a white and British perspective anyway) is the recognition that what was considered to be consigned to the imperial past, very much lives on in the present. Offering a critique of liberal capitalism, Bookchin writes, '[a]s long as liberal environmentalism is structured around the social status quo, property rights always prevail over public rights and power always prevails over powerlessness' (1989, p. 15), whilst simultaneously observing that planned communist and socialist economies, that are also founded on industrialism and economic growth, are just as capable of ecological destruction. It is from these critiques of existing statist political systems that Bookchin arrives at advocating for political education, citizens assemblies, libertarian municipalism, and the formation of ecocommunities. This remaking of democracy at a local and city level, with sensitivity shown to the limits of the natural world to meet human needs, offers a well-developed political methodology through which to 'overcome the social and ecological consequences of the centralized state, modern market economies, and the technologies they spawn' (Light, 1998a, p. 8). For Bookchin, it is only at the scale of the city (defined as a municipal area as opposed to a megalopolis), rather than at the level of the individual or the state, that such political ambitions can come to full fruition.

Differentiation and diversity, of species and of the forms that societies and civilisations experiment with, is important to social ecology. It is perceived that the appearance of greater and greater differentiation is a primary outcome of biological evolution, and thus the differentiation and diversity of human culture becomes one expression of that evo-lutionary principle. A distinction is made by Bookchin between first nature and second nature, where first nature is those biological forms and processes that proceed the appearance of the second nature of human cultures, civilisations, and social structures. Crucially, the dom-ination of nature by humans has its origins in how humans dominate each other, and not the other way around, with the source of that urge to dominate being located by Bookchin at the transition point between nomadic and settled societies and the need for older and materially unproductive members of the community to maintain their existence through the hoarding of wealth and knowledge (Bookchin, 2015).

Bookchin is especially critical of deep ecology, accusing it of easily slipping into an anti-human Malthusian perspective that all too easily becomes co-opted by racists and fascists in the form of eco-fascism. For example, the refrain that the climate crisis can be addressed through reducing population growth, without acknowledging the great varia-tion in levels of consumption and emissions between people of different countries or different economic groups. Bookchin is just as critical of the overt spiritualism that frequently seeps into deep ecology, worry-ing that it both leads to muddled hedonism, irrational thinking, and the simple reformulation of hierarchies, observing that '[t]he moment human beings fall to their knees before anything that is "higher" than themselves, hierarchy, will have made its first triumph over freedom, and human backs will be exposed to all the burdens that can be inflicted on them by social domination' (1989, p. 13). A reliance upon spiritual-ity and religion, or upon subjective and emotive responses, to address social injustices and ecological catastrophe, is not enough and needs to, at the very least, be tempered with reference to what can be ration-ally and objectively observed within history, political theory, and col-lective experience. For Bookchin, this is because '[w]hat is clear is that human beings are much too intelligent not to have a rational society; the most serious question we face is whether they are rational enough to achieve one' (2015, p. 30). This recourse to the power of rationality reflects Bookchin's defence of Enlightenment and humanist principles. Importantly, from an art therapy perspective, Bookchin offers a cau-tion against believing that psychotherapy, or any other form of personal transformation, alone will address the social and ecological problems faced. It is only the systemic transformation of society, and its fixation on hierarchies, competition, and profit, that will prevail.

Whilst social ecology is helpful in terms of joining together environ-mental and social processes, a critique of social ecology, from a deep ecology perspective, is that it does not present a nuanced enough under-standing of actual other-than-human processes. And that it perpetu-ates the assumption that the other-than-human can be manipulated and controlled for human benefit – albeit with mutual benefits that are shared equally between human and other-than-human beings. Once again adopting an Enlightenment and humanist position, Bookchin presents human consciousness and human culture as being at the apex of evolution, proposing that humans should strive to be fully conscious and reflexive stewards of nature through the rational directing of evolutionary processes. Bookchin has also been critiqued for relying both on very narrow anthropological examples and very limited historical and archaeological evidence to support his arguments about the emergence of hierarchies within early human settled societies and cities, of over-emphasising the cooperative and collaborative aspects observed within the natural world, and of being too dogmatic in his unwillingness to compromise his utopian political vision (Light, 1998b, Price, 2012). Whilst these criticisms are valid, what social ecology offers is a solid body of thought, and imaginary potential, as to how to form a bridge between a practical and rational political praxis that is founded upon the political principles of social justice, participatory democracy, and municipalism, and the many forms of ecological desires and concerns that are expressed physically, emotionally, and spiritually.

Traditional ecological knowledge

Where the three preceding ecologies are disseminated primarily via the written form, and are articulated mostly in the language of academia and political discourse, traditional ecological knowledge – or indigenous knowledge and native science as it is also referred to as – whilst possessing its own academic tradition of dissemination, is primarily an oral tradition that contains observations gathered over many generations, whilst also creating meaning through the use of story and allegory. However, not being part of an easily identifiable indigenous culture with its own long history of ecological wisdom passed from one generation to the next, I have had to rely primarily on its written form to gain some understanding of its many teachings. Outside of the rather vague warning given to me as a child by my mother about not picking dandelions because they can make you wee, there is little that I have gained about traditional ecological knowledge in my own upbringing. In adulthood, I did learn that the leaves of dandelions, if ingested, are actually mildly diuretic, so that warning does make some sense, even if my mother was just repeating a folktale that she had been taught as a child. This lack reflects my urban upbringing on the edges of London. I imagine that had my parents been keener gardeners or foragers then I might have rather more ecological knowledge that was traditional in nature, assuming that they in turn had been introduced to such knowledge by their parents or wider family and community. But they, and their own parents, also had an urban upbringing, working in factories, shops, and offices. I have to go back seven generations on my father's side to the 18th century to find a written record of relatives who lived and worked on the land as yeomen farmers. At some time in the middle of the 19th century, John Lofts (five generations past) moved from Little Downham, in rural East Anglia to Bethnal Green, East London. This, I assume, reflects the general drift of working people from the country to the city as part of the industrialisation of Britain at that time. Any traditional knowledge of how to tend and farm the land has been long forgotten by my family, along with those stories and songs that would have transmitted that knowledge. All of which is to say that if my understanding of the ecological knowledge that emerges from my own tradition, history and culture, is limited, it is even more so of those traditions that are far removed from my own. This is especially the case, given how traditional ecological knowledge is presented as knowledge that is gained, developed, and shared through participation of the whole person being immersed within a place-based community of humans and other-than-humans. As Gregory Cajete notes, '[t]o understand the foundations of Native Science one must become open to the roles of sensation, perception, imagination, emotion, symbols, and spirit as well as concepts, logic, and rational empiricism' (2018, p. 16). This way of forming and gaining knowledge resonates with the arts-based methodologies I am familiar with, and Chapter 2 will draw particular attention to imagination and emotion as valid epistemologies within those methodologies.

As would be expected, there are many expressions of traditional and indigenous ecological knowledge, which reflects both its long history and the great diversity of points of origin. There are though some commonalities between them that Dan Shilling (2018) identifies. These are:

- Reciprocity and respect the bond between all members of the land family.
- Reverence toward nature plays a critical role in religious ceremonies, hunting rituals, arts and crafts, agricultural techniques, and other day-to-day activities.
- One's relationship to the land is shaped by something other than economic profit.
- To speak of an individual owning land is anathema, not unlike owning another person, akin to slavery.
- Each generation has a responsibility to leave a healthy world to future generations.

(p. 12)

These common themes speak to the formation and maintenance of a strong bond between people and the land. It is apparent that each of those commonalities present challenges to the cultural paradigms that dominate modern western thought (Narvaez, 2021). Shared ownership and valuing that which is not of economic worth or that cannot be turned into power and status, being especially challenging. In addition to these themes, there are other shared features of traditional ecological knowledge that I think are worth noting here. The first of these is how time is conceived differently within scientific and indigenous knowledge, or rather how there is a difference between the western science conception of time being linear and always flowing like a river in one consistent direction, and the many other ways in which time is conceived within different traditions. For example, the past and the present being in front of a person and therefore visible, whilst the future is behind and invisible, as perceived by the Aymara speakers of South America. Or, the Anishinaabe view of time being cyclical, in which past, present, and future generations walk through life simultaneously. Ancestral knowledge and consideration for one's descendants go hand in hand, and this is reflected in the last of the commonalities listed above. Time is therefore more akin to a lake than a river in this understanding. Incorporating different conceptions of time is one crucial example of the importance of opening up ways of knowing in order to expand understanding beyond purely modern and empirical traditions. In response to recording indigenous knowledge holders understanding of time, it has been concluded that '[a]wareness of differences in temporal constructions of knowledge is essential for cross-epistemological sharing, for maintaining respect across knowledge holders, and for seeing climate change as it really is' (Chisholm Hatfield et al., 2018, p. 9). This has implications for working with the emotional components of climate change, and for making use of imaginal and arts-based methods, in terms of being sensitive to the relationship between the past, present, and future in how people and communities tell stories of change and adaptation, and for taking account of traditional knowledge, even where such knowledge might sit beneath more recent ways of knowing.

The second theme, and one that aligns closely with the first commonality above, is the theme of kinship between the human and the other-than-human. Writing from the perspective of the Rarámuri people of Mexico, Enrique Salmon, uses the concept of *iwigara* to introduce the idea of kincentric ecology (Salmon, 2000). Iwigara 'channels the idea that all life, spiritual and physical, is interconnected in a continual cycle' (p. 1328), so that humans, other-than-human beings, land, air, and water, are all considered to be related, and to all share the same breath. This forms a fundamental set of believes on which all aspects of Rarámuri life draw upon. As Salmon observes '[i]t is iwigara that guides agriculture, medicine, and foraging. The use of plants for healing and for food offers a fundamental relationship from which the Rarámuri view themselves as participants in their natural community' (p. 1329). Examples show how this set of principles leads to a relationship with plants, animals, and the land that approaches the use of those from a position of caretaking and enhancing, rather than one of exploitation and extraction. Robin Wall Kimmerer, an enrolled member of the Potawatomi Nation, writes eloquently of how similar doctrines and codes from her own tradition translate into the practice of the Honourable Harvest (Kimmerer, 2020). It advocates for, amongst other things, seeking permission before taking, not taking the first or the only example, taking only what is needed and is given, giving thanks, and giving back. The Honourable Harvest is 'reinforced in small acts of daily life' (p. 183). The notion of reciprocity between the human and the other-than-human is central to the Honourable Harvest. There is a sense of humility and an acceptance of the interconnections and interdependence of things and beings, and a very different notion of what sustainability means when land, animals, and plants are understood to be kin.

The echoes of traditional ecological knowledge are to be found in the three other ecologies already described. The expanded view of time, in which the past, the present, and the future coexist and are intimately related resonates with the mediations upon the coexistence of different times scales within dark ecology. The veneration and honouring of all beings as kin appears just as strongly within deep ecology. The intimate role of humans in the care for nature, and the Honourable Harvest, have their parallels within the way that social ecology envisions the mutually beneficial relationship between the human and the other-than-human.

There is a critique to be made that introducing traditional ecological knowledge in this way (especially by someone such as myself who is not a holder of such knowledge) is itself an act of colonisation, that it comes close to a form of appropriation, and that it has a romanticised view of both nature and the way in which humans interact with it. I would accept this criticism. The lure of taking traditional ecological knowledge out of its historical, geographic, and political context, as part of a process of magical thinking that fantasises about it being an easy solution to climate crisis that can be adopted by anyone, anywhere, without acknowledging historical and ongoing injustices and subsequent acts of indigenous resistance, and without a consideration of the need for material reparations, can be strong. This is especially true if adopting only the spiritual components of traditional ecological knowledge – something that Bookchin is particularly cautious about – as it bypasses the material aspects of hunting, fishing, harvesting, farming, and the raising of children, that form such a core component of traditional ecological knowledge. Despite these caveats, it is necessary to acknowledge the existence and very real importance of traditional ecological knowledge, simply because it does form both a major part of many peoples' existing worldview, and is arguably the foundation upon which more contemporary and western science-based ecological worldviews, as well as European Enlightenment ideals of freedom and liberty (Mann, 2012;

Graeber and Wengrow, 2021), are built upon. It is also a body of knowledge that may well become the most pertinent for the times ahead.

Ecologies combined

How do these differing and overlapping ecologies combine within my own practice of social action art therapy? In synthesising elements of the ecologies presented, it means gaining a fuller appreciation of the historical and political context of any given piece of ecological knowledge. It means gaining a fuller understanding of colonial history and its links to the exploitation of people and planet. It means acknowledging trauma – the trauma of the loss of species, loss of land, of the continuing effects of colonialism. It means, as Vanessa Andreotti frames it, recognising the broken house and poisoned metabolism of modernity, and being prepared to go beyond, beneath, and outside of the idea that modernity can be fixed or saved (Andreotti et al., 2015; Andreotti et al., 2018). It means, in the words of Timothy Morton, being playfully serious, so as to not always make rational sense and to embrace different ways of experiencing and knowing the world – or rather experiencing and knowing a plurality of different worlds. It means always being conscious of the need to go beyond my own perspective – to acknowledge the experiences of humans of other places and times, and the experiences of other-than-humans. If following the teaching of traditional ecological knowledge, it means living that knowledge by being conscious of my actions upon the land and of how I fit into a long chain of beings. In Chapter 2, where I outline the features of social action and social justice art therapy, the place and role of ecologies within those will become apparent where there is an exploration of how art therapy can and does incorporate more than the intrapsychic into its ways of being.

Outline of chapters

Chapter 2 brings together an outline of what social action art therapy entails – including its close relationship with social justice art therapy – alongside an introduction to ecotherapy and those arts therapies that incorporate attention to the natural environmental. Chapter 2 also includes an overview of arts-based research methodologies. It is assumed that the majority of readers will be familiar with the main tenets of art therapy and art psychotherapy such as the use of art as a metaphor, the role of the image within the therapeutic relationship, and the place of transference and counter-transference. As such, those aspects of art therapy are not dwelt upon in detail. Instead, I show how aspects of psychology, social justice, and ecology can be synthesised within therapeutic and research contexts in which art takes a central position. This does mean pushing at the boundaries of both theory and practice in order to find ways to address intersecting social, political, and ecological crises. A fundamental boundary, and the attendant hierarchy that it sets up, which is pushed at and challenged, is the one that defines the difference between the human and the other-than-human. This boundary is however representative of other boundaries and hierarchies that are indicative of contemporary thought: the boundary between reason and emotion for example, or the one between science and art.

One way of framing and making sense of those boundaries and hierarchies is to consider how they have been constructed by modernity. Modernity within this context refers to those philosophies and values that underpin science and politics within contemporary western and industrialised civilisations, and which have been in ascendancy over the last four to five hundred years. Whilst the seemingly abstract topic of modernity is not the usual focus of art therapy, Chapter 3 spends time articulating those features of modernity that I consider are most pertinent to social action art therapy. Those features are to do with the way in which modernity is presented as a system that favours human reason above all other ways of knowing, at the same time as its defines the pinnacle of humanity as being predominantly white and male and relegates to the margins and makes subterranean all that is not deemed logical or rationale, or too emotional, or not human enough. Despite this, what is relegated to the margins constantly re-emerges in hybrid and metaphorical forms. The work of Bruno Latour (Latour, 1993) and Bolivar Echeverría (Echeverría, 2019), who explore these aspects of modernity, and question if we have ever been modern or are perhaps not modern enough, is referenced in this discussion of modernity. Part of what marks modernity out as a dominant philosophy is how it creates a hierarchy of epistemologies and ontologies, where empiricism and the scientific process as way of understanding and directing both what it defines as human – society, politics, economics – and what it defines as nature – biology, chemistry, physics – are placed above other forms of knowing and being. As a counter point to this hierarchy is the bringing to the fore ways of knowing and being that highly value the body, place, emotions, and stories. These can especially be found within both art therapy and arts-based research. They are also central to two sets of ideas that I and others have found essential to working with the topics of refuge and migration, domestic violence and abuse, and climate crisis. These are belonging and imagination. Belonging, within contemporary sociological and political practice, is presented as an emotional attachment to a feeling of being at home and of being safe, both in the present and in the hoped for future (Yuval-Davis, 2011). Home is both a physical and a psychic place and can be as attached to landscape as it can to dwellings. For example, in discerning what belonging means for refugees and asylum seekers, the central role of community and geographical place in the formation of a sense of belonging emerges

(O'Neill, 2010). Alongside belonging, imagination plays a fundamental role within how I have used art therapy and arts-based research to address social action and social justice. Imagination is an epistemology that takes into account the physical, emotional, and political elements of the construction and enactment of knowledge. A feminist understanding of imagination is a helpful way of drawing together those elements; in particular, the way in which feminist-standpoint theory centres lived experience and views all knowledge as being situated both in time and in place. Imagination, in the form of going beyond one's own situated position, along with attentive listening and observation, is required when responding to the call to make the starting point of any enquiry into the lived experience of other people (Harding, 2004). If the ecologies introduced above are brought into focus here, especially traditional ecological knowledge, that call extends outwards to incorporate the lived experience of other-than-human people.

It is argued that climate change is both a consequence and a defining feature of modernity (Andreotti et al., 2015) and of whiteness (Akomolafe, 2020), where domination, colonisation, and extraction are the primary political and economic motivators that structure many contemporary civilisations. This argument states that the violence that is inflicted by humans upon other-than-humans and other humans comes from the same paradigm. As such, I propose that understanding responses to other moments of crisis, such as seeking refuge from political, economic, or domestic violence, and any subsequent process of recovery, offers lessons that can be applied to imagining how to respond and adapt to climate change, which itself can be considered to be another form of violence. Chapter 4 is therefore devoted to presenting and illustrating how I have used the principles of social action art therapy, and arts-based research, when working with people who have sought refuge from political violence and those who have sought refuge from domestic violence and abuse. Images and words from both projects are presented, with notions of belonging and the formation of transitional stories that emerge in this context preparing the way for thinking about working with climate crisis. Essential to understanding the nature of political and domestic violence is gaining a better understanding of how violence works in general. With this in mind, Chapter 4 opens with an exploration of conceptions of violence that are useful to consider within the contexts explored in this and the following chapters, which focus on social action art therapy in response to climate crisis. This includes the notion of slow violence – a conception of violence used by Rob Nixon (Nixon, 2011), exposing how environmental damage disproportionately effects those places and peoples least able to resist it over sustained periods of time.

Bringing together the theoretical and the practical elements of the preceding chapters, the use of social action art therapy to address the emotional components of climate crisis is the focus of Chapter 5. Examples, including visual images, are provided of the development of a way of working in three different contexts: environmental activism; higher education; and diverse communities. Within the workshops that have been conducted so far, a wide range of feelings have been expressed in response to considering climate change and crisis; feelings that include anger, despair, guilt, hopelessness, helplessness, and isolation. Participants have used visual mediums, music, and movement to explore those and other feelings in more detail. The focus moves from the individual to the collective, recognising the power of collective responses to climate crisis. What frequently arises as an outcome of participation is a sense of people not being so isolated, and of the feelings that are expressed being validated and normalised. Where it feels appropriate, participants are invited to imagine how the communities and organisations they are located within might adapt to climate change and transition towards something different. Whilst there is the appearance of imagined solutions that might mitigate the impact of climate change in the present, there is more often an expression of ideas and feelings that offer ways of preparing for, and living with, the consequences of a change climate. To help other art therapists adopt and develop these ideas further within those contexts and communities that they know best, example workshop plans are provided as an appendix.

In concluding this book, I restate the case for the use of a social action approach to art therapy, which is informed by and parallels a social justice approach, in response to different forms of crisis. Those crises are framed as emerging from aspects of modernity, and I repeat the observations made about the structure and limits of modernity, drawing attention to how the violence that modernity enables disrupts belonging. One violence that modernity enables, and that is central to its continued existence, is the violence of suppression and exclusion – of people, of ideas, of landscapes, of futures – that do not fit with the fundamental belief in its own supremacy as a system of thought. A way of addressing the consequence of that violence, and the attendant disruption to belonging and to possible alternative and diverse futures, is to use creativity and imagination to consider other ways of being in the present and in the future. What creativity and imagination bring to that objective is a different epistemology to the dominant epistemology of modernity; one that places knowledge that is embodied and poetic on a par with that which is drawn from reason and empiricism.

A fundamental formula that is returned to throughout this book is that there can be no meaningful response to climate crisis without equally responding to social injustices. The formula, as I interpret it, also has an implicit focus upon collective responses to injustices and crisis. With that formula in mind, the lessons gained from working in an arts-based way with the injustices of migration, asylum, and domestic violence and abuse, provide an appropriate foundation for addressing how climate crisis impacts both belonging and how the future is imagined in a collective and communal way. Where the books ends is to state that social action art therapy can bring people together to address collectively the emotional components of climate crisis, and in turn to imagine how they can individually and collectively make the transition to a future that has love and care at its centre.

Notes

1 https://data2.unhcr.org/en/situations/mediterranean [accessed: 5/1/2022]
2 https://www.theccc.org.uk/2020/04/21/how-much-more-climate-change-is-inevitable-for-the-uk/ [accessed: 30/9/2020]

References

Akomolafe, B. 2020. *I, coronavirus. Mother. Monster. Activist.* [Online]. Available: https://bayoakomolafe.net/project/i-coronavirus-mother-monster-activist/ [Accessed 31/12/2020].

Andreotti, V. O., Stein, S., Ahenakew, C. & Hunt, D. 2015. Mapping interpretations of decolonization in the context of higher education. *Decolonization: Indigeneity, Education & Society* 4, 21–40.

Andreotti, V. O., Stein, S., Sutherland, A., Pashby, K., Susa, R. & Amsler, S. 2018. Mobilising different conversations about global justice in education: toward alternative futures in uncertain times. *Policy and Practice: A Development Education Review*, 26, 9–41.

Atkins, S. S. & Snyder, M. A. 2018. *Nature-Based Expressive Arts Therapy: Integrating the Expressive Arts and Ecotherapy.* London; Philadelphia, PA: Jessica Kingsley Publishers.

Bonneuil, C. & Fressoz, J.-B. 2017. *The Shock of the Anthropocene: The Earth, History, and Us.* London: Verso Books.

Bookchin, M. 1989. *Remaking Society.* London: Black Rose Books.

Bookchin, M. 1993. *Deep Ecology and Anarchism: A Polemic.* London: Freedom Press.

Bookchin, M. 2015. *The Next Revolution: Popular Assemblies and the Promise of Direct Democracy.* London: Verso Books.

Cajete, G. 2018. Native Science and Sustaining Indigenous Communities. *In:* Nelson, M. K. & Shilling, D. (eds.) *Traditional Ecological Knowledge: Learning from Indigenous Practices for Environmental Sustainability.* Cambridge: Cambridge University Press.

Chakrabarty, D. 2009. The climate of history: four theses. *Critical Inquiry*, 35, 197–222.

Chisholm Hatfield, S., Marino, E., Whyte, K. P., Dello, K. D. & Mote, P. W. 2018. Indian time: time, seasonality, and culture in traditional ecological knowledge of climate change. *Ecological Processes*, 7, 25.

Crutzen, P. J. 2002. Geology of mankind. *Nature*, 415, 23.

Echeverría, B. 2019. *Modernity and "Whiteness".* Cambridge: The Polity Press.

Estes, N. 2019. *Our History Is the Future: Standing Rock Versus the Dakota Access Pipeline, the Long Tradition of Indigenous Resistance.* London: Verso.

Fox, W. 1995. *Towards a Transpersonal Ecology: Developing New Foundations for Environmentalism.* Totnes: Resurgence.

Graeber, D. & Wengrow, D. 2021. *The Dawn of Everything: A New History of Humanity.* London: Penguin.

Hall, S., Critcher, C., Jefferson, T., Clarke, J. & Roberts, B. 1978. *Policing the Crisis: Mugging, the State, and Law and Order.* London: Macmillan.

Harding, S. 2004. *The Feminist Standpoint Theory Reader: Intellectual & Political Controversies.* London: Routledge.

Heginworth, I. S. 2009. *Environmental Arts Therapy and the Tree of Life.* Exeter: Spirit's Rest.

Heginworth, I. S. & Nash, G. (eds.) 2019. *Environmental Arts Therapy: The Wild Frontiers of the Heart.* London: Routledge.

IPCC. 2018. Summary for Policymakers. *In:* Global Warming of 1.5°C. An IPCC Special Report on the impacts of global warming of 1.5°C above pre-industrial levels and related global greenhouse gas emission pathways, in the context of strengthening the global response to the threat of climate change, sustainable development, and efforts to eradicate poverty [Masson-Delmotte, V., P. Zhai, H.-O. Pörtner, D. Roberts, J. Skea, P.R. Shukla, A. Pirani, W. Moufouma-Okia, C. Péan, R. Pidcock, S. Connors, J.B.R. Matthews, Y. Chen, X. Zhou, M.I. Gomis, E. Lonnoy, T. Maycock, M. Tignor, and T. Waterfield (eds.)]. Geneva, Switzerland: World Meteorological Organization.

Kimmerer, R. W. 2020. *Braiding Sweetgrass: Indigenous Knowledge, Scientific Knowledge and the Teachings of Plants.* London: Penguin Books.

Krishnamurti, J. 1992. *On Nature and the Environment.* London: Victor Gollancz Ltd.

Latour, B. 1993. *We Have Never Been Modern.* New York: Harvester Wheatsheaf.

Lewis, S. & Maslin, M. 2018. *The Human Planet: How We Created the Anthropocene.* London: Verso.

Light, A. 1998a. Introduction: Bookchin as/and Social Ecology. *In:* Light, A. (ed.) *Social Ecology after Bookchin.* New York: The Guilford Press.

Light, A. (ed.) 1998b. *Social Ecology after Bookchin.* New York; London: Guilford.

Lorde, A. 2018. *The Master's Tools Will Never Dismantle the Master's House.* London: Penguin Modern Classics.

Mann, C. C. 2012. *1491: New Revelations of the Americas Before Columbus.* New York: Knopf.

Masson-Delmotte, V., P. Zhai, A., Pirani, S. L., Connors, C., Péan, S., Berger, N., Caud, Y., Chen, L., Goldfarb, M. I., Gomis, M., Huang, K., Leitzell, E., Lonnoy, J. B. R., Matthews, T. K., Maycock, T., Waterfield, O., Yelekçi, R. & Yu, A. B. Z. E. 2021. *Climate Change 2021: The Physical Science Basis. Contribution of Working Group I to the Sixth Assessment Report of the Intergovernmental Panel on Climate Change.* Cambridge: Cambridge University Press.

Mcconnell, A. 2020. *The Politics of Crisis Terminology.* London: Oxford University Press.

Mcewan, K., Giles, D., Clarke, F. J., Kotera, Y., Evans, G., Terebenina, O., Minou, L., Teeling, C., Basran, J., Wood, W. & Weil, D. 2021. A pragmatic controlled trial of forest bathing compared with compassionate mind training in the UK: impacts on self-reported wellbeing and heart rate variability. *Sustainability*, 13, 1380.

Morton, T. 2013. *Hyperobjects: Philosophy and Ecology after the End of the World.* Minneapolis, MN: University of Minnesota Press.

Morton, T. 2016. *Dark Ecology: For a Logic of Future Coextistence.* New York: Columbia University Press.

Næss, A. 1990. *Ecology, Community and Lifestyle: Outline of an Ecosophy.* Cambridge: Cambridge University Press.

Narvaez, D. F. 2021. Colonial psychology: The psychology we all recognize [Online]. *Psychology Today.* Available: https://www.psychologytoday.com/gb/blog/moral-landscapes/202107/colonial-psychology-the-psychology-we-all-recognize [Accessed 6/12/2021].

Nixon, R. 2011. *Slow Violence and the Environmentalism of the Poor.* Harvard: Harvard University Press.

O'Neill, M. 2010. *Asylum, Migration and Community.* Bristol: The Policy Press.

Price, A. 2012. *Recovering Bookchin: Social Ecology and the Crises of Our Time.* Norway: New Compass Press.

Richardson, M., Hunt, A., Hinds, J., Bragg, R., Fido, D., Petronzi, D., Barbett, L., Clitherow, T. & White, M. 2019. A measure of nature connectedness for children and adults: validation, performance, and insights. *Sustainability,* 11, 3250.

Ruddiman, W. F. 2005. *Plows, Plagues, and Petroleum: How Humans Took Control of Climate.* Princeton, NJ: Princeton University Press.

Salmon, E. 2000. Kincentric ecology: indigenous perceptions of the human-nature relationship. *Ecological Applications – ECOL APPL,* 10, 1327–1332.

Shilling, D. 2018. Introduction: The Soul of Sustainability. *In:* Nelson, M. K. & Shilling, D. (eds.) *Traditional Ecological Knowledge: Learning from Indigenous Practices for Environmental Sustainability.* Cambridge: Cambridge University Press.

Spratt, D. & Dunlop, I. 2018. *What Lies Beneath: The Underestimate of Climate Risk.* Melbourne: National Centre for Climate Restoration.

Yuval-Davis, N. 2011. *The Politics of Belonging: Intersectional Contestations.* London: Sage.

2 Social action art therapy, ecotherapy, and arts-based research methods

This chapter weaves together three different sets of ideas and practices that form a coherent foundation for framing a way of working with crisis. The chapter begins by presenting an outline of social action art therapy, including its relationship to social justice and social change, as well as to art therapy and art psychotherapy. Reference is made to Francis Kaplan's (Kaplan, 2005; Kaplan, 2007) pioneering work on social action therapy, and Savneet Talwar's (Talwar, 2019a) development of art therapy for social justice, drawing out the commonalities and differences between them. The incorporation of political and social contexts into psychologically focused thought and practice is the key element of social action art therapy that is expanded upon here. Existing ecological thought within art therapy is examined where it appears in the form of *environmental art therapy* and *nature-based expressive arts therapies*. Looking beyond art therapy, the growing body of literature from an ecopsychology and ecotherapy perspective, which advocates for attention to the unconscious aspects of responses to ecological crisis, and the parallel call for psychotherapists to account for external social and political realities in their work, is reviewed. Reference is made to the work of Joseph Dodds (2011), Renée Lertzman (2015), and others who are contributing to the work of the *Climate Psychology Alliance*.

In this chapter, I also provide an outline of various arts-based research methods, exploring how they synthesise with social action art therapy to create a way of working that has the potential to be transformative and emancipatory for those who participate. Paying attention to the unconscious is carried on here when thinking about research methods that seek to go beyond purely cognitive responses to the questions that researchers seek to answer. The multi-layered, messy, and poetic quality of the arts lend themselves well to enabling the articulation and interpretation of other-than-cognitive responses. The arts also allow a natural emergence of objects and places within expressions of the real and the imagined, the rational and the irrational. The role of subjectivity, reflexivity, and intersectionality within the research methods advocated for is expanded upon.

DOI: 10.4324/9781003142560-2

When writing about social action art therapy in 2007, and wondering if art therapy could tolerate the inclusion of attention to social forces, Dan Hocoy asked the important question '[h]ow can art therapy maintain its identity and be so flexible?' (2007, p. 33). Whilst the question is no less valid now, it has become easier to give an affirmative answer because of the expansion in thinking that has taken place around the issues of a socially and politically engaged form of art therapy. This same process can be observed in other therapies, and within psychology more generally. Since that question was first asked by Hocoy, a number of things have taken place that make it much harder to *not* pay attention to society and politics upon the interior lives of clients: economic shock, demands for racial justice, climate, and ecological crisis.

Social action art therapy

Art therapy has a long enough history to have developed different modalities and approaches that are of value within a range of community and clinical contexts. The intention here is not to provide a complete and comprehensive overview of the history art therapy as that objective has been addressed elsewhere (Waller, 1991; Hogan, 2001; Potash, 2005; Junge, 2010; Stepney, 2019). Nor is there an intention to outline here the range of philosophies and theories that underpin the various approaches within contemporary art therapy and art psychotherapy. What I am concerned with, instead, is to draw together evidence that supports the case for the use of an approach to art therapy that takes as much interest in the shared social and political components of lived experience as it does to the psychological components of individuals and families. This is an approach to art therapy that is frequently referred to as social action art therapy, and that has very close associations to the framing of art therapy as social justice, and the expressive arts therapies for social change. Social action, social justice, and social change frequently appear as interchangeable terms within the art therapy literature.

Social action and social justice, as art therapy approaches, would appear to have a stronger history within the United States than elsewhere, with US-based art therapists Dan Hocoy (Hocoy, 2005; Hocoy, 2006; Hocoy, 2007), Frances Kaplan (Kaplan, 2005; Kaplan, 2007), and Savneet Talwar (Talwar, 2010, Talwar, 2019a, Talwar, 2015, Talwar, 2003) being key proponents of the use of art therapy to directly address social concerns. From a European perspective, via the European Graduate School in Switzerland, there is the development of *expressive arts therapies* to enact social change (Levine and Levine, 2011). Ephrut Huss has developed a strong tradition of using art in therapeutic and social change contexts within Israel, Sri Lanka, and Bedouin communities (Huss, 2013; Huss et al., 2016; Huss et al., 2018). There are examples of a socially focused art therapy in many different context, including work with refugees in Calais (Lloyd et al., 2018), exploring imaginatively responsible play as an alternative to neo-liberalism (Landers, 2012), and employing a feminist approach to better understand birth trauma (Hogan, 2020)

Social action, social justice, and social change all share a view that health, illness, and healing are shaped as much by social and political factors as they are by individual and interpersonal experiences, and in practice they take account of the collective and communal nature of health, illness, and healing. The simplest way of explaining this is to say that sociological and psychological explanations of suffering and well-being have equal worth. They also share an explicit aim of using the arts to effect change at a social and community level as well as at the individual and interpersonal level. By paying attention to the biographical experiences of people and communities, there is within each a desire to give voice to what is usually marginalised, and to produce knowledge that contributes to social justice and participatory democracy (O'Neill and Harindranath, 2006). With reference to asylum and migration, social researcher Maggie O'Neill (2008) proposes that '[t]he right to speak, be heard and recognized are central aspects of "social justice" and feed in to cultural politics' (p. 44). Before proceeding to consider in more detail how social action, social justice, and social change appear within the context of art therapy, it is worth commenting on the different terms *art therapy* and *expressive arts therapies* as they appear here. There is more that unites them than separates them. The terms can be interchangeable to some extent; in the same way that social action, social justice, and social change are. The main difference being that art therapy is more likely to adopt the language of psychotherapy, neurology, and attachment. Art therapy, like music therapy, dance therapy, or drama therapy, also tends to focus on the use of just one art form. Expressive arts therapies have a somewhat looser association to psychotherapy and are more likely to integrate different art forms into their practice. Differences in terms can also reflect variations in training and professional regulations between countries and states. My own preference here is to use the term art therapy, as that best reflects my own training and practice within a UK context.

Introducing the idea of social action art therapy, Francis Kaplan proposes that '[w]e cannot separate the people we treat from the cultural settings in which they live and by which they have been influenced. None of us exists in a social vacuum; each of our psyches comprises a unique amalgam of genetic endowment, family upbringing, environmental influences, and collective history' (Kaplan, 2005, p. 2). Whilst reference to social justice is of greater significance in more recent literature, it does appear in earlier literature outlining social action art therapy. For example, Dan Hocoy (2007) writes that 'art therapy as social action might have one invariable telos or endpoint in mind – that of achieving just and peaceful human communities' (p. 34). Deborah Golub (2005) also provides a perspective that points towards social justice when they write that social action art therapy is 'a participatory, collaborative process that emphasizes artmaking as a vehicle by which communities name and understand their realities, identify their needs and strengths, and transform their lives in ways that contribute to individual and collective well-being and social justice' (p. 17). Kaplan in a dialogue with Nisha Sajnani (Sajnani and Kaplan, 2012) about the interplay between social action and social justice states that she thinks of 'social action as a means of achieving social justice, something to be worked toward as a long-term goal and as a condition in which change for the betterment of society has been firmly established' (p. 166).

The awareness of individuals and communities not being isolated objects existing in vacuums, rather being dynamic subjects within a process of relationships, is fundamental to social action art therapy. This framing of the individual as embedded within a wider social context is also a fundamental feature of art therapy for social justice. Hocoy (2007) visualises the relationship between the individual and society within the context of art therapy as three interconnected circles. These represent society, the client, and the therapist. Each of those circles contains a multitude of dominant and marginalised voices. The objective here is to draw attention to the creation of a space 'where multiple voices, equal in status, are continually in dialogue and permeable to reciprocal influence' (p. 34). The overlapping of the individual and society, and the attention to other voices, is, as shall be seen below, just as fundamental to ecopsychologies, and to broader forms of ecology. When starting to incorporate an ecological perspective into this model of art therapy, around these three circles can be added a larger circle to represent an ecological sphere within which the three human-centred circles of society, client, and therapist coexist within the other-than-human sphere. The multitude of voices that Hocoy alludes to then starts to include the other-than-human, which opens pathways to accommodating other types of knowledge and experience into the therapeutic encounter; something that ecotherapies and ecopsychologies value especially.

Whilst art therapy for social justice and social action art therapy share many features, one difference is that there tends to be a stronger critique of art therapy's adoption of a modernist epistemology from a social justice perspective (Talwar, 2019b), as well as a more explicit critique of the faults lines within capitalism and neo-liberalism. Savneet Talwar builds their approach to art therapy for social justice upon an understanding of the consequences of collective and historical trauma, stating that art therapists 'need to consider how representations of race, ethnicity, class, gender, sexuality, disability, and religion bring into the present the intergenerational trauma of the past, as represented by slavery, violence, patriarchy, heteronormativity, economic and class-based oppression, ableism, and other forms of systemic oppression' (2015, p. 101). This difference in focus between social action and social justice, as they appear within art therapy literature, is a possible consequence of the social justice literature appearing after the financial crisis of 2008; a crisis that exposed the weaknesses of the neo-liberal version of capitalism. It is also a consequence of how a social justice approach to art therapy adopts intersectionality as a way of thinking about the relationship between individuals and society (Talwar, 2010, Talwar, 2019a). First developed by Kimberley Crenshaw (Crenshaw, 1989; Crenshaw, 1991) to explain why legal statutes that seek to address race discrimination do not automatically lead to an improvement in opportunities and access, intersectionality argues that race is one amongst other aspects of identity and social belonging that come together to create social hierarchies and experiences of discrimination. Crenshaw (1989) was initially interested in how the experience of Black women was marginalised within feminist discourse as it emerged within legal proceedings. Focusing on race or gender in isolation misses the complexity of their interaction as a whole and how that shapes experience. The challenge put forward is that '[n]either Black liberationist politics nor feminist theory can ignore the intersectional experiences of those whom the movements claim as their respective constituents' (p. 166). Intersectionality is a significant component of the contemporary understanding of race and racism, and has expanded to include class, age, sexuality, and physical and mental abilities. There is therefore, within an approach that adopts an understanding of intersectionality, a focus on broader social structures that work to maintain hierarchies and discrimination. This includes addressing the economic models that currently dominate and intersect with aspects of identity and social belonging. It is this explicit analysis of economics and race that marks social justice out as being positioned differently to social action.

Reflexivity and privilege

Art therapy, like all psychological therapies, is founded upon the idea that the therapist, and the relationship that they have with clients and patients, is as crucial to the work as the techniques and methods employed. The two become indistinguishable at a certain point. Transference and countertransference are likely to be the most relevant examples of the therapeutic relationship that art therapist will be familiar with. Art therapists will likewise be familiar and comfortable with self-reflection being an essential element in creating a good therapeutic relationship. What a social action approach advocates for is the widening out of that act of self-reflection so that it incorporates social and political influences, in addition to personal and familial influences. The Black Lives Matter movement, and expressions of anger and pain in response to the murder of George Floyd in early 2020, has accelerated this need for art therapists, especially those who are white, to consider their own role within patterns of colonialism and racial oppression.

Hocoy (2005) provides the example of homophobia to illustrate oppression in action; how, within the history of psychiatry, homophobia appears within the pathologising of sexualities that do not conform to a heterosexual definition of appropriate and healthy. Whilst some older ideas about sexual deviation have fallen away, their echoes remain in transphobia and ambivalence about different sexualities. Where one version of gender and sexuality is privileged, other versions become marginalised. In response, art therapists are asked to consider '[w]hom or what in society does art therapy privilege or serve?' (p. 8). Hocoy suggests that these ideas have real implications for art therapists: recognising and responding to our own internalising of social injustices; committing to addressing those social injustices at a local and global level where we can; developing a sensitivity to the reciprocal relationship between the personal and the political, the psychological and the social. This perspective draws upon an understanding of how social and cultural values become internalised within individuals. From a depth psychology perspective there is an inescapable interconnection between internal mental processes and the external physical and social world. This interconnection flows both ways, such that '[i]ndividual and collective experiences and actions cocreate one another in a reciprocal field' (p. 10). Interconnectivity, and reciprocal relationships between the individual and the collective at a human level, can be seen to parallel how interconnectivity between the human and the other-than-human is framed within those ecologies introduced in Chapter 1.

From the perspective of the expressive arts therapies for social change, the observation is made by Stephen Levine that, through the process of becoming more mainstream, art therapy has become risk adverse and lost some of its original radical edge and willingness to challenge mainstream psychiatry (Levine, 2011). Levine suggests that this has led to some art therapists moving into other fields, such as the expressive arts therapies, in order to continue a practice that is critical of dominant forms of psychological care. Talwar (2019b) also observes that art therapy has become increasingly medicalised and neurological in its focus, as well as being rather too reliant upon a psychology that has a history of producing reductive narratives of deviancy and normality. Susan Hadley (2013) argues that art therapists need to learn to recognise dominant narratives that lead to oppressive practice, as well coming to acknowledge their own privilege, if they are to contribute to the causes of social justice. The need to examine privilege is also deemed to be a crucial element of art therapists' response to social and political trauma if working from a social justice perspective (Karcher, 2017). There is an emphasis on the need for the art therapist to address their own relationship with oppressive and unjust social forces, how those forces become voiced through the therapist, and to be introspective, reflexive, and curious about the appearance of those forces within conscious and unconscious processes. If attention is not given to the influence of those forces, then art therapists run the risk of repeating and amplifying harmful social norms and biases within their work.

Whatever term is used – social action, social justice, or social change – the argument I would wish to make is that there is a requirement to pay close attention to the reciprocal interactions between individual and social processes. The understanding that art therapists already have about being reflective and sensitive to their own internal sensations, thoughts, and feelings is expanded out to include their place within communal, social, and political relationships. And, as repeated frequently, the further step is to include sensitivity towards the relationships that are kept with the other-than-human. It is this later aspect that I now turn to in outlining ideas and practices within ecotherapy and ecopsychology, which in turn leads to considering the emergence of environmental and nature-based art therapy, and its associations with social action and social justice.

Ecotherapy and ecopsychology

References to nature, the environment, and the relationship between the human and other-than-human are not new to psychology or to psychologically informed therapies. There is though a growing and explicit attention to how they might contribute to ecological and climate crisis. This includes responding therapeutically to the mental and emotional suffering that comes from either the direct experience of environmental destruction, or the witnessing of it from a distance. It also includes using psychological insights to better understand what helps and what hinders individuals, organisations, and governments from taking action to limit the impact of climate change, or to prepare for its effects. There is a common desire to reexamine the foundations of whatever theory or practice is being considered in light of ecological insights. This is found in Thomas Doherty's (2016) provision of a clear and inclusive starting point for thinking about what ecotherapy is. For Doherty, ecotherapy is any psychotherapeutically aligned activity that is 'undertaken with an ecological consciousness or intent' (p. 14) and that 'welcomes ecological aspects of self, identity and behaviour into the psychotherapeutic arena' (p. 15). It also seen in Mary-Jane Rust's (2020) observation that the 'central narrative of ecopsychology is that we once knew we were part of the web of life – physically, psychologically, and spiritually – and in the course of our long history we have become increasingly disconnected from the rest of nature' (p. 52). As was presented in Chapter 1, this story of disconnection and separation, of humans being once deeply embedded and inseparable from an organic environment, but now increasingly inhabiting an artificial environment that has been sculpted and manufactured *by* humans *for* humans, is one that is observable across many versions of ecological thought and practice. It is therefore no surprise to see that insight gain credibility within psychological therapies.

If separation is one essential component of ecological thought, and its subsequent appearance within therapy, the corresponding counter narrative is the need to reconnect. This reconnection is powerfully expressed in the call to be wild, or to re-wild various internal and external human spaces. Thus, gestalt psychotherapist, Steffi Bednarek (2019), wonders if the psychotherapies should be willing to imagine and embrace a wilding, even a re-wilding, of their practice if they are to respond to this time of crisis. She writes that '[w]idening our field of psychotherapy may therefore need to include practices which move us beyond the story of a separate self, practices which explore nonordinary states of consciousness, and nature-based practices that transcend a sense of separation from the world and our anthropocentric perspective' (p. 11). The wilding that Bednarek advocates for includes going outside – both literally and in the sense of going beyond the current orthodox traditions that underpin therapeutic practice. For example, it includes going beyond the individual to think about the communal and social aspects of experience. Increasingly, it includes a consideration of the other-than-human as equal parts of those. This aspect of psychotherapy made wild aligns with a social action and social justice approach to art therapy, where there is an encouragement to move beyond the individual. The notion of re-wilding, from a psychological perspective, was advocated for early on by James Hillman. His proposition is that the soul, the mind, every encounter, and every place be approached in the same way that a protected and conserved physical landscape is approached. We are encouraged to tread lightly and to 'come to a more psychological notion of wilderness following the definition inherent in the rules governing wilderness areas: enter and enjoy but make no mark. Disturb nothing, leave no trace – if possible, not even a footprint' (Hillman and Morre, 1989, p. 104). Recourse to organic processes in the metaphor of the re-wilding of the mind, of the soul, and of therapy has parallels in those references to metabolism and composting as metaphors for how new growth can emerge from old and discarded memories and histories (Andreotti et al., 2018), and of how the relationship between the human and other-than-human has mycelium-like qualities to it in terms of hidden but vital threads reaching out beneath the surface.

The suffering identified as being related to a disconnection from nature, and to the pressing issue of climate crisis, comes in the form of anxiety, grief, or various types of trauma responses. Eco-grief, eco-anxiety, vicarious trauma, and pre-traumatic stress disorder have been suggested as ways of categorising these feelings. But there is the criticism that this takes a reductionist approach and feeds into a narrative of curing symptoms and repairing the individual, rather than tackling the social and collective causes of the symptoms (Bednarek, 2019). It is in attempting to address that reductionist approach to emotional suffering that re-wilding and treading lightly appear as appealing metaphors for how to be with the feelings that climate crisis evokes. Those feelings of grief and anxiety can be framed as a normal and healthy response to a disconnection with nature, to real threats posed by ecological crisis, and to whole societies acting in suicidal ways (Cunsolo et al., 2020). They can also be re-framed as a necessary expression of empathy for the other-than-human, which is especially apparent in children and young people (Sharp and Hickman, 2019; Hickman et al., 2021). Loss appears as a frequent catalyst for these responses. This includes not only loss in the present, but also imagined and predicted loss in the future. And whilst the future is made extremely uncertain by climate crisis, an argument is made from a psychoanalytic perspective that 'the first move must be to start telling the truth about loss. We need to withdraw the projections of loss from the future and make loss real in the present' (Randall, 2009, p. 125). This is especially pertinent for those communities in the prosperous Global North who have so far been protected from the most egregious impacts of climate change, such as floods, fires, crop failures, and water shortages. Each passing year makes this projection of loss into the future harder to maintain though. A particular expression of environmental loss and grief, *solastalgia*, refers to the painful feelings of disruption that occur when a person's or a communities' sense of belonging towards an environment is adversely affected by ecological damage and violence (Albrecht, 2005). The relationship between solastalgia, belonging, and violence is a relevant one in the context of my own thinking about social action art therapy and crisis, where crisis refers to asylum, domestic violence and abuse, and environmental damage. Each of those crises are a form of violence that disrupts the relationship between a person and the place called 'home,' where home is a singular physical dwelling, a diffuse set of locations within an environment, or kinship relations with the human and the other-than-human.

From a psychoanalytic perspective, there is attention to how knowledge and experience of climate crisis triggers emotional responses that are related back to early infancy and childhood. As well as the anxiety and grief identified above, there is the appearance of defensive positions such as scepticism, denial, and ambivalence. The detachment of the human from nature is seen as a parallel to the psychoanalytic idea of splitting, where there is an association of the 'good' with self and the 'bad' with what is not self. This process operates at an individual and at a social level (Dodds, 2011). Many of us might claim that we agree wholeheartedly with the existence of climate crisis but still find ways to sidestep its reality or respond in ways that might limit our choices as consumers (Dodds, 2019). This insight has important implications for how communication and action take place between people and how political mobilisation can proceed. Instead of a simplified dichotomy of good and bad, a more nuanced third position that acknowledges the pain and our limited ability to deal with its causes appears. Using Kleinian terminology, this is akin to moving from a paranoid-schizoid position to a depressive position, which from an ecological position 'involve[s] mourning for the losses involved in environmental destruction, guilt for the damage done and a reparative drive to restore, repair, and recreate the lost and damaged world' (Dodds, 2011, p. 69). Such insights lead to several suggestions about approaches to communication. Splitting, and the attendant behaviours of denial and projection, can be reduced by being careful to frame communication about climate and ecological crisis in ways that do not deliberately, or inadvertently, provoke shame and guilt (Lertzman, 2015). At the very least, an acknowledgment of the appearance of shame and guilt has a value if wanting to avoid retreats into cynicism and despair. Paying careful attention to feelings of fear, anxiety, loss, and ambivalence is increasingly advocated for by environmental activists and organisations attempting to influence individual behaviour and political policies. One of *Extinction Rebellion's* biggest contributions is how it has legitimatised and allowed feelings of grief and anger within environmental campaigning. The *Climate Psychology Alliance* in the United Kingdom has led the way on the development of 'climate cafes,' where people are able to come together to share those strong emotional responses to climate crisis that are not always easy to name and be present with. The rationale being that sustainable ecologically minded action that is based on hope and courage is more likely to take place when difficult or painful feelings are neither repressed nor projected (Hamilton, 2019).

Writing from a dialogical and hermeneutic position, psychoanalyst Donna Orange makes a powerful and profound case for psychoanalysis engaging fully with both climate crisis and social injustices, presenting them as intimately linked (Orange, 2017). As with Bednarek (2019), there is an urgency to the call for therapists to use their insights and skills to acknowledge the crisis and to affect change. Orange debates that a radical ethical approach is required to truly grasp and respond to what confronts us – an 'us' that is addressed to those with privilege and power – so that all lives are equally valued and that we learn to see clearly the links between our own choices and the impact upon the lives of others. The thinking of Emmanuel Levinas and Paul Ricoeur about our relationships and obligations to each other leads Orange to sate her belief that 'only a radical ethics of the fundamental worth of every human life will make the difference we need in the climate crisis' (2017, p. 120). To this position, Orange adds the common ecological attention to posthumanist empathy, in which the other-than-human is included in contemplations of the 'other.'

Ecotherapy and ecopsychology offer then a helpful set of concepts that can complement existing art therapy theory and practice. Like the social justice and social action strands of art therapy, there is a willingness to challenge how the relationship between the individual and society is framed. There is a desire to question modern and western conceptions of human psychology in light of ecological insights. Chief amongst these insights is that the other-than-human is increasingly allowed an equal voice within the consideration of what being human entails.

Environmental and nature-based arts therapy

The influence of ecological insights and thought upon therapeutic practice extends into art therapy. Whilst a sensitivity to the appearance of nature within the practice of art therapy has been present at the level of thinking about its appearance within imagination and images for some time (Case, 2005), there is a growing interest in adopting an explicitly environmental approach to framing and practicing art therapy. *Environmental arts therapy* has emerged within the United Kingdom as a set of ideas and practices around which those art therapists who are interested in the environment have coalesced, with arts therapist Ian Heginworth doing much to articulate this approach. Starting in November, and the time of the Gaelic festival of Samhain, Heginworth leads the reader through a slow yearlong cycle of poetic meditations and rituals that borrow heavily from imagined Celtic traditions, and which are combined with acts of creative (Heginworth, 2009). The cycle is a metaphorical one that emphasises birth, growth, death, mourning, and rebirth. November is presented as a time of preparing for the winter months, where a physical connection to hawthorns, fungi, the bark of birch trees, and leaf fall, draws attention to the fruitfulness of the season that has been, and which is now being composted to feed and make space for the return of the new. One activity that is suggested by Heginworth involves lying down in a pile of leaves in a posture that represents an old aspect of the self that is to be left behind, and allowing that self to be covered over with more leaves. We are asked to sink down and imagine dissolving into the ground, before rising up again and wondering at the shape left behind in the fallen leaves. In December, attention moves further into thoughts about a descent into shadows and darkness. The rowan tree is presented as a manifestation of the Tree of

Life within the abyss. Further allusions are made to Lilith from Judaic mythology and her archetypal association with the 'dark feminine,' which, according to Heginworth, represents 'our feeling response to the wounds that make us who we are. It settles in the pits and dungeons of the self, in the harsh and barren wastes within' (p. 32). The call is made to enter this dark place, to acknowledge it, and to learn from it.

Allusions to the dark feminine reflect a frequent association made between nature and the feminine. This is an association that requires further explanation as it is one that appears in ecology generally, and specifically in other writings exploring how the arts therapies can work in ways that are sensitive to ecology and nature (Heginworth and Nash, 2019a). When appearing in this context, the feminine is positioned in relationship with the masculine in ways that are used to contrast feeling and intuition with reason and cognition, or the wild with the tamed. The comparison rests upon Carl Jung's theory of *anima* and *animus* and the supposed indigenous conceptions of Mother Earth (Edinburgh, 2020). Heginworth retells the story of Adam and Eve from the Christian tradition, noticing that '[t]he story tells us that we lose our place in the garden because of our pursuit of knowledge, our relationship with the masculine' (2009, p. 23). This interpretation is then associated with violence and abuse against women and children, the destruction of natural habitats, and ultimately 'the neglect and abuse of the feeling self within' (p. 23). Whilst there is much merit in considering the ways in which varying forms of knowledge and experience are valued within different epistemologies, ontologies, and traditions, there is also a need to be mindful of not conflating too quickly the way the concept of the feminine and the masculine, in the context of how they appear within ecological thought or in how they are used as a metaphor for different forms of knowing, with the biological characteristics of sex or the way in which gender is socially defined. As Latour and Lenton (2019) caution when observing the gendering of the mythological figure of Gaia, '[a]ny look at Hesiod will show that there is nothing maternal, womanly, or even godly in such a dangerous, archaic, cunning, and chthonic figure that precedes all the gods' (p. 166).

In contrast to positive associations of the feminine with the Earth and nature, Genevive Lloyd critiques how the division of the male and the female within western philosophy, from Francis Bacon to Simone de Beauvoir, is used to diminish both the value of the emotional and sensual, and the contribution of women to science, philosophy, and politics (Lloyd, 1993). Lloyd draws attention to how the dominance of men over women in the social and political sphere has been used to justify the domination of nature by scientific reason and logic, where women are considered to be more closely associated to nature and the irrational than men are. A similar critique is made in considering the miss-conceptualising of nature-culture relationships in how indigenous cultures are interpreted and represented within western anthropology (Strathern, 1980). There are no consistent or universal dichotomies of male-female, man-women, or nature-culture within the anthropological or archaeological record. Rather, there are shifting hierarchical relationships between evolving and situated meanings. As such, western and modern ideas about the division between culture-nature and their association with male-female cannot be imposed onto other cultures or other times. Whilst such metaphors and associations might be useful in helping to ground complex and the ephemeral processes within physical forms, there is a need to be mindful of how those are historically situated, and how they just as easily contribute to the construction and maintenance of hierarchies. A central tenet in ecological thought and practice is that many dualisms are constructions of thought that are in need of re-imagining. Thus, the terms spacetime, bodymind, and inter-being appear frequently within ecological texts in attempts to challenge binary positions linguistically. The existing dualisms of man-woman, female-male, and feminine-masculine require a similar re-imagining in the context of ecological thought and environmental practice. At the very least, we need to think about why those terms have the meaning they do in contemporary thought, and if we wish to subscribe to those meanings or challenge them. Queer ecology and trans ecology offer a useful commentary here about challenging and transcending such binaries (Clare, 2009).

The ideas and practices developed by Heginworth have led to the offering of an environmental arts therapy programme in the United Kingdom (Heginworth and Nash, 2019b), where it is defined as being 'an arts-based approach to working therapeutically in outdoor spaces and emerges from the creative exchange that has occurred between the ecopsychology movement and the arts therapies professions and communities' (p. 2) to which is added the understanding that the 'therapeutic combination of the arts and nature, human and other-than-human, is informed by a growing awareness and interest in the work of ecopsychology which considers our interdependency and interrelationship with the Earth' (p. 2). Again, reconnection with nature is framed as a fundamental alternative to the story of alienation and separation between the human and the other-than-human that an ecological perspective sees as endemic in contemporary societies and cultures. In terms of how environmental arts therapies relate to other models of art therapy, there is an appreciation of theories of attachment and to how natural objects and places can act as transitional objects within environmental arts therapy (Ponton, 2019). There is also in environmental arts therapy much consideration given to the safe holding of clients' feelings, and their creative expressions, when working away from standard therapeutic settings. This examination of safety has echoes with the challenges encountered when taking art therapy into refugee camps and when responding to natural disasters (Lloyd et al., 2018).

A similar initiative to environmental arts therapy can be found in the development of *nature-based expressive arts therapy* at the Appalachian State University, US, and the European Graduate School, Switzerland (Atkins and Snyder, 2018). Interestingly, this is the same European Graduate School that has been a catalyst for the development of art therapy for social change that is introduced above (Levine and Levine, 2011). Sally Atkins and Melia Snyder adopt a story-based approach to the presentation of ideas and practices related to scientific, philosophical, artistic, and indigenous understandings of nature and ecology, whilst making a frequent reference to the concept of *rhizomes* (Guattarri, 2014) to imagine how ideas emerge and grow in organic and often hidden ways as a result of shifting non-linear relationships between each other.

Echoing a social justice approach to art therapy, there is within nature-based expressive arts therapy an explicit critique appears of capitalism and its associations with conquest, exploitation, and domination. As noted earlier, the appearance of this criticism of capitalism within a contemporary arts therapy context reflects a growing dissatisfaction with the dominant economic system, which has flowed from the economic crisis of 2008. Atkins and Snyder also observe how many therapies, and therapists, have been co-opted into the medicalised and evidence-based approach to suffering and healing, with attention being drawn to the limitations of orthodox medical model and psychological models to deal with how the ecological crisis impacts human health. This is an observation that suggests a need for sort of re-wilding of therapy alluded to within the psychotherapies (Bednarek, 2019). The most unique feature of nature-based expressive therapies, and the one that I find of most relevance to my own ecological thought and practice, is its critical attention to the appearance of different epistemologies within the arts therapies. The examination of epistemologies points to the sort of fundamental shift in thinking and being that climate crisis demands. Three epistemologies, or ecoepistemologies, are proposed: an epistemology of the sacred, an epistemology of the senses, and an epistemology of the intimate. An epistemology of the sacred refers to an understanding of the world and universe as full of sentient beings and subjects, that exist is a state of reciprocity and mutual exchange, with humans as just one part of that whole. This epistemology challenges the idea of human domination and superiority over nature. Within an epistemology of the senses that domination of nature is presented as a result of the valuing of mental reason and rationality over more body-centred forms of perception. This draws upon an idea of embodiment where space is made for the pre and non-verbal aspects of perception and being in engagement with the world. This is also an epistemology that is central to an appreciation of the value of arts-based research that I present later in this chapter. Intimacy is an epistemological position that questions the boundaries of the self when we come to consider our relationship with other life forms or natural processes; the trillions of bacteria cells within the human body for example, or our place within the carbon cycle through the act of breathing. Each of these three epistemologies challenges the distinction between self and not-self, and between human and non-human. Each of them challenges the primacy of the dominant paradigms and epistemologies of modernity, including a challenge to what being human means.

Addressing climate and ecological crisis directly, Atkins and Snyder (2018) make a powerful case for how arts therapists can use their knowledge and skills to respond to these crises. They write that '[t]his is our call and our response/ability as nature-based expressive artists – to claim and use the medicine of the arts and the Earth in the service of all life' (p. 134), adding that '[w]e allow ourselves to be moved by what we experience, engaging directly with the world around us in a way that furthers beauty, sustainability and wellbeing for all life' (p. 135). References to service and wellbeing for all life are an indication of how a concern for the natural environment can incorporate a concern for human and social wellbeing. The aligning of the use of the arts therapies for social and ecological justice with reference to beauty takes on the language of an epistemology of the sacred. This use of sacred language is perhaps most evident in how indigenous and traditional knowledge and wisdom is co-opted into thinking about the environment. Whether these are the words of *Woman Stand Shining* (Pat McCabe) of the Dine people, North America (Edinburgh, 2020), lessons from the Quechua people of South America (Atkins and Snyder, 2018), or reference to Celtic rituals (Heginworth, 2009), there is the suggestion that contemporary secular and industrial societies can learn from cultures and peoples with traditions that have a more balanced and reciprocal relationship with nature. There is the suggestion that in doing so, arts therapists can engage with the sort of sacred and active hope that activist and group facilitator Joanna Macy promotes (Macy and Johnstone, 2012) in addressing various global crises.

To recap then, environmental arts therapy and nature-based expressive arts therapy offer helpful foundations for considering how to use art therapy for the benefit of addressing the climate and ecological crisis. They are both able to demonstrate that it is possible to work safely as an art therapist within outdoor settings. They both draw upon those fundamental features of ecological thought that is also evident within ecotherapies and ecopsychologies: the wilding of therapy; the re-connection with nature; the equal valuing of the human and the other-than-human. Each of these features is enhanced by the introduction of creativity and imagination, and the use of ritual. Both environmental arts therapy and nature-based expressive arts therapy attempt to learn from traditions of thought and ritual practice that either pre-date or run parallel to secular and modern perceptions of the individual, society, and of nature. Environmental arts therapy in particular draws heavily upon mythologies and rituals that have been associated with contemporary interpretations of Celtic tradition and culture. This attention to traditions of thought and practice that incorporate bringing the care of that which is beyond the individual self – society and ecology – into focus provides a helpful point of contact between environmental and nature-based art therapy, and the principles of social actions and social justice.

Arts-based research

The final part of this chapter presents those features of arts-based research that I have found helpful in my own research, and that complement those aspects of social action art therapy which I have already outlined. I have participated in the use of arts-based methods to understand experience of migration and asylum, to understand the experience of transitioning away from domestic abuse, and to understand emotional responses to knowledge of climate crisis. The results of those investigations, and their synthesis with social action art therapy, are expanded upon in Chapters 4 and 5. The aspect of arts-based research that is most relevant, in the context of advocating for a social action and social justice approach to art therapy, is its closeness to participatory and emancipatory approaches to research within the social sciences and the humanities. Of note is how arts-based research aligns with how imagining new and more just futures, in addition to uncovering and reflecting present lived experiences, are valid concerns for what has been termed *new paradigm research*. Such research 'will criticize how things are and will imagine how they could be different' (Denzin, 2000, p. 262). New paradigm research refers to the methodological response to the 'crisis of representation' within sociology end ethnography, which is itself a response to the uncertainties and anxieties about claims of universal truths within contemporary western culture. If an appreciation of the plurality of truths is of greater significance than the identification of singular universal truths then the embracing of multiple voices and metaphors that the arts allow is an appropriate way to conduct such research. Susan Finley (2003) identifies three key commitments to new paradigm research: 'first, to deep participant and researcher interactions and involvements; second, to professional, personal, and political actions that might improve participants' lives; and third, to future-oriented work that is based in a visionary perspective that encompasses social justice, community, diversity, civic discourse, and caring' (p. 282). These new forms aim to widen the scope of research in terms of who can participate, how people participate, and what actions emerge from that participation. In addition, positionality, reflexivity, community, voice, and reciprocity are, Finley points out, all standards of new paradigm qualitative research. Positionality and reflexivity refer to the need for researchers to be aware of how they are situated within society and how that shapes their privilege, power, and subsequent relationship with research participants and the knowledge that they share. I have found intersectionality to be a useful way of framing and navigating the development of that awareness. The intention is to be critical of power dynamics within research in order to create more egalitarian forms of knowledge. Thus, the emphasis upon the voice of the participant or the community, and the formation of reciprocal relationships between those doing research and those being researched. Frequently, participants become co-designers and co-conductors of research. This is not without its challenges in terms of whose voice is most dominant in a given context. New methods of dissemination have democratised the sharing of research, but there is still a strong academic hierarchy in place when it comes to access to research resources and channels of dissemination.

When using arts-based research methods to better understanding women's experiences of domestic violence and abuse, a feminist version of arts-based research became necessary. Claims about the potential of a synthesis between arts-based methods and feminist-standpoint theory have been made by arts-based researcher Patricia Leavy (2007) who suggests that the use of the arts within research can serve the aims of feminism in general through making visible subjugated voices, the promotion of affect as a valid form of knowledge, and engaging with women's imagination. Leavy points out that many feminist researchers reject positivist claims to represent the truth about social life, arguing that positivism 'is based on several dichotomies including: objective-subjective, rational-emotional, researcher-researched, mind-body, and fact-fiction. Many feminists have theorized that this perspective on the research process contributes to the kind of scientific practices that have oppressed women and other minorities' (p. 2). Leavy suggests that in response to the criticisms made about the dichotomies inherent within a positivist epistemology, feminist-informed researchers have developed methodologies that focus on collaboration, reflexivity, and attention to subjugated perspectives. Fiction, imagination, narrative, and autobiography are presented as a means of providing alternative and visionary interpretations and representations of social life, whilst embodiment is offered as a way of addressing the mind-body dichotomy that is evident within positivist thinking.

The imaginative and visionary qualities of arts-based research contribute to what I believe make it a radical and appropriate response to crisis. Elsewhere, in thinking about health-related research, I have argued that because arts-based research sits comfortably with uncertainty and ambiguity, it provides a method of working with those topics, and people, that are easy to ignore, turn away from, or remain ignorant about (Bird, 2022). Within the medical humanities, ethnography, and sociology, there is a long-standing interest in reaching a fuller understanding of what it means to be healthy, sick, and to engage with healing practices. Iain Wilkinson makes the claim that all sociological works are in some way concerned with the causes and consequences of suffering (Wilkinson, 2004), arguing for an overt aim of bringing to light suffering and injustice in order to bring researchers, participants, and audiences closer to one another. This intimacy aids civic compassion and human rights; features that Wilkinson identifies as foundational, though often neglected, objectives of modernity. As I will explore more fuller in Chapter 3, modernity values rationality and empiricism above all other forms of knowledge, but if it is to stay relevant in a world of multiple and intersecting global crises (ecological, social, economic), whilst also meeting the objective of emancipation and widening rights (for the human and the other-than-human), it needs to gather to itself other sorts of knowledge, and it needs to accommodate different epistemologies and competing forms of explanation (Latour, 1993). As an example of this in action, Stuart Wood (2020) uses music to understand the post-verbal world of dementia, and makes direct reference to how ethnography and the medical humanities are leaning more upon creative methods to access and interpret those experiences that are not easily verbalised or rationalised. Wood does however make the observation that '[t]he move from the unspeakable to the attempt to name is not a simple epistemological line' (p. 75). The epistemology that underpins arts-based research is one that favours interpretation, intuition, and imagination as much as, if not more than, it values hypothesis, analysis, and rationality. This gives space for the ambiguous and the awkward. The arts are in general comfortable with the ineffable, and being in a state of uncertainty. Arts-based research makes an attempt to use those qualities to help interpret and translate the ineffable elements of experience. That it always fails to do this in a way that forecloses any alternative analysis of the data, is not a weakness, but rather an expression of how it embraces expressions of diversity and plurality. From the perspective of art therapy, this is a manifestation of being comfortable with the making of mess; whilst from a perspective somewhat outside of art therapy – that of posthumanist literature – this expresses a willingness to enter into the places of shadows, where monsters and tricksters dwell (Akomolafe, 2020).

The specific elements of arts-based research that I identify as justifying the label radical are: addressing social marginalisation; the role of creative expression in the co-production of knowledge; the potential transformative benefits of research participation; moving beyond words to access those epistemologies that value emotional, intuitive, imaginative, and embodied responses to questions. Addressing social marginalisation and the co-production of knowledge are features that are similar to what helps to define social action and social justice, and what appears within new paradigm research. The element concerned with the transformative aspect of arts-based resonates with an 'ethics of care' approach to arts-based methods in which there is an explicit acknowledgment that it works for the good of the participating individual or groups (Wiles et al., 2011). An ethics of care stresses that researchers ought to aspire to practice reflexivity, whilst taking account of the situated and place-based nature of knowledge and their own privileged position within the production of knowledge. An ethics of care is also a helpful way to navigate institutional concerns about the benefits of participation and co-production. What makes arts-based research unique is the aspect related to the use of different epistemologies. This element fits with aspects already identified about using alternatives to rationality and empiricism within social action, ecological thought and the reassessment of modernity. This element will have relevance throughout Chapter 3, when thinking through how belonging, imagination, and modernity relate to responding to crisis. Because of the coming together of these elements within arts-based research, I maintain that the radical nature of arts-based research is a necessary and valid way of approaching times of crisis and uncertainty. Especially so now, where climate change brought about by global heating creates feelings of doubt and anxiety about the relationship between the human and the other-than-human, and prompts a reimagining of our relationship to history and progress (Chakrabarty, 2009; Morton, 2013).

Summary

What has been put forward in this chapter is a network of concepts that I have found helpful in my own development as an art therapist in the time, and the communities, that I have found myself living and working within. Throughout that development, there has been a weaving together of art therapy as a psychotherapeutic intervention, art therapy as one component in the move towards social justice and change, and the use of art-based research methods as another component. These have helped me to work with people classified as refugees and asylum seekers, and with people transitioning away from domestic violence and abuse. This has involved working in both an explicitly therapeutic capacity and as a part of academic research projects. At points, research and therapeutic objectives have worked in parallel, and the careful and considered synthesis of those ideas presented in this chapter was required to manage the joining together of those objectives. With a growing desire to better understand the emotional impact of climate change, in response to my own struggles, gaining an appreciation of the influence of ecology upon psychological and psychotherapeutic thought and practice, as well as its incorporation into the arts therapies has been beneficial. There is a good enough fit between social action art therapy, ecological thought, and art-based research to make me believe strongly that together they can form a helpful response to this particular time of crisis. It is unrealistic to suggest that there is a single feature that unites them, but there is a commonality to be found in the desire to go beyond theoretical boundaries in the search for ways to respond more fully to the world of the human and the other-than-human. In the case of social action art therapy, this means pushing at the boundaries of professional definitions and practice by bringing psychological and political insights together. Something similar occurs within ecopsychotherapy with the joining together of psychological and ecological insight, where there is a willingness to consider how ideas like wholeness and interbeing can contribute to thinking and acting differently. The importance of this observation will become clearer in Chapter 3, where the influence of modernity is considered in detail, alongside the concepts of imagination and belonging.

References

Akomolafe, B. 2020. *I, Coronavirus. Mother. Monster. Activist.* [Online]. Available: https://bayoakomolafe.net/project/i-coronavirus-mother-monster-activist/ [Accessed 31/12/20].

Albrecht, G. 2005. Solastalgia: a new concept in human health and identity. *Philosophy Activism Nature*, 3, 41–44.

Andreotti, V., Stein, S., Sutherland, A., Pashby, K., Susa, R. & Amsler, S. 2018. Mobilising different conversations about global justice in education: toward alternative futures in uncertain times. *Policy and Practice: A Development Education Review*, 26, 9–41.

Atkins, S. S. & Snyder, M. A. 2018. *Nature-Based Expressive Arts Therapy: Integrating the Expressive Arts and Ecotherapy.* London & Philadelphia: Jessica Kingsley Publishers.

Bednarek, S. 2019. 'This is an emergency' – proposals for a collective response to the climate crisis. *British Gestal Journal*, 28, 4–13.

Bird, J. 2022. Arts-Based Research as a Radical Methodology Within Healthcare. *In:* Hinsliff-Smith, K., Mcgarry, J. & Ali, P. (eds.) *Arts Based Health Care Research: A Multidisciplinary Perspective.* London: Springer.

Case, C. 2005. *Imagining Animals: Art, Psychotherapy and Primitive States of Mind.* London: Routledge.

Chakrabarty, D. 2009. The climate of history: four theses. *Critical Inquiry*, 35, 197–222.

Clare, E. 2009. *Exile and Pride: Disability, Queeness, and Liberation.* Durham: Duke University Press.

Crenshaw, K. W. 1989. Demarginalizing the intersection of race and sex: a black feminist critique of antidiscrimination doctrine, feminist theory and antiracist politics. *University of Chicago Legal Forum*, 1(1).

Crenshaw, K. W. 1991. Mapping the margins: intersectionality, identity politics, and violence against women of color. *Stanford Law Review*, 43, 1241–1299.

Cunsolo, A., Harper, S. L., Minor, K., Hayes, K., Williams, K. G. & Howard, C. 2020. Ecological grief and anxiety: the start of a healthy response to climate change? *Lancet Planet Health*, 4, e261–e263.

Denzin, N. K. 2000. Aesthetics and the practices of qualitative inquiry. *Qualitative Inquiry*, 6, 256–265.

Dodds, J. 2011. *Psychoanalysis and Ecology at the Edge of Chaos*. London: Routledge.

Dodds, J. 2019. Otto Fenichel and ecopsychoanalysis in the anthropocene. *Psychoanalytic Perspectives*, 16, 195–207.

Doherty, T. J. 2016. Theoretical and Empirical Foundations for Ecotherapy. *In:* Jordan, M. & Hinds, J. (eds.) *Ecotherapy: Theory, Research and Practice*. London: Palgrave.

Edinburgh, M. 2020. Bringing the Outside In: Reflecting upon Mother Within a Pilot Group in Environmental Arts Therapy. *In:* Heginworth, I. S. & Nash, G. (eds.) *Environmental Arts Therapy: The Wild Frontiers of the Heart*. London: Routledge.

Finley, S. 2003. Arts-based inquiry, QI: seven years from crisis to guerrilla warfare. *Qualitative Inquiry*, 9, 281–296.

Golub, D. 2005. Social action art therapy. *Art Therapy*, 22, 17–23.

Guattarri, F. 2014. *The Three Ecologies*. London: Bloomsbury Academic.

Hadley, S. 2013. Dominant narratives: complicity and the need for vigilance in the creative arts therapies. *The Arts in Psychotherapy*, 40, 373–381.

Hamilton, J. 2019. Emotions, Reflexivity and the Long Haul: What We Do About How We Feel About Climate Change. *In:* Hoggett, P. (ed.) *Climate Psychology: On Indifference to Disaster*. Switzerland: Palgrave Macmillan.

Heginworth, I. S. 2009. *Environmental Arts Therapy and the Tree of Life*. Exeter: Spirit's Rest.

Heginworth, I. S. & Nash, G. (eds.) 2019a. *Environmental Arts Therapy: The Wild Frontiers of the Heart*. London: Routledge.

Heginworth, I. S. & Nash, G. 2019b. Introduction by the Editors. *In:* Heginworth, I. S. & Nash, G. (eds.) *Environmental Arts Therapy: The Wild Frontiers of the Heart*. London: Routledge.

Hickman, C., Marks, E., Pihkala, P., Clayton, S., Lewandowski, E. R., Mayall, E. E., Wray, B., Mellor, C. & Van Susteren, L. 2021. Climate anxiety in children and young people and their beliefs about government responses to climate change: a global survey. *Lancet Planet Health*, 5, 863–873.

Hillman, J. & Morre, T. 1989. *A Blue Fire: The Essential James Hillman*. London: Routledge.

Hocoy, D. 2005. Art therapy and social action: a transpersonal framework. *Art Therapy: Journal of the American Art Therapy Association*, 22, 7.

Hocoy, D. 2006. Art therapy: working in the borderlands. *Art Therapy*, 23, 132–135.

Hocoy, D. 2007. Art Therapy as a Tool for Social Change: A Conceptual Model. *In:* Kaplan, F. (ed.) *Art Therapy and Social Action*. London: Jessica Kingsley Publishers.

Hogan, S. 2001. *Healing Arts: The History of Art Therapy*. London: Jessica Kingsley Publishers.

Hogan, S. 2020. Birth shock! What role might arts engagement have to play in antenatal and postnatal care? *Journal of Applied Arts & Health*, 11, 239–254.

Huss, E. 2013. *What We See and What We Say: Using Images in Research, Therapy, Empowerment, and Social Change*. London: Routledge.

Huss, E., Braun-Lewensohn, O. & Ganayiem, H. 2018. Using arts-based research to access sense of coherence in marginalised indigenous Bedouin youth. *International Journal of Psychology*, 53, 64–71.

Huss, E., Kaufman, R., Avgar, A. & Shuker, E. 2016. Arts as a vehicle for community building and post-disaster development. *Disasters*, 40, 284–303.

Junge, M. B. 2010. *The Modern History of Art Therapy in the United States*. Springfield, IL: Charles C Thomas.

Kaplan, F. F. 2005. What is social action art therapy? *Art Therapy*, 22, 2–2.

Kaplan, F. F. (ed.). 2007. *Art Therapy and Social Action*. London: Jessica Kingsley Publishers.

Karcher, O. P. 2017. Sociopolitical oppression, trauma, and healing: moving toward a social justice art therapy framework. *Art Therapy*, 34, 123–128.

Landers, F. 2012. Urban play: imaginatively responsible behavior as an alternative to neoliberalism. *The Arts in Psychotherapy*, 39, 201–205.

Latour, B. 1993. *We Have Never Been Modern*. New York: Harvester Wheatsheaf.

Latour, B. & Lenton, T. 2019. Extending the domain of freedom, or why Gaia is so hard to understand. *Critical Inquiry*, 45, 659–680.

Leavy, P. 2007. Merging Feminist Principles and Art-Based Methodologies. *American Sociological Association Annual Conference*. New York.

Lertzman, R. 2015. *Environmental Melancholia*. London: Routledge.

Levine, E. G. & Levine, S. K. 2011. *Art in Action: Expressive Arts Therapy and Social Change*. Philadelphia, PA: Jessica Kingsley Publishers.

Levine, S. K. 2011. Art Opens to the World: Expressive Arts and Social Action. *In:* Levine, E. G. & Levine, S. K. (eds.) *Art in Action: Expressive Arts Therapies and Social Change*. London: Jessica Kingsley Publishers.

Lloyd, B., Press, N. & Usiskin, M. 2018. The Calais Winds took our plans away: art therapy as shelter. *Journal of Applied Arts & Health*, 9, 171–184.

Lloyd, G. 1993. *The Man of Reason; 'Male' & 'Female' in Western Philosophy*. London: Routledge.

Macy, J. & Johnstone, C. 2012. *Active Hope: How to Face the Mess We're in Without Going Crazy*. Novato, CA: New World Library.

Morton, T. 2013. *Hyperobjects: Philosophy and Ecology after the End of the World*. Minnesota: University of Minnesota Press.

O'Neill, M. 2008. Transnational refugees: the transformative role of art? *Forum Qualitative Sozialforschung/Forum: Qualitative Social Research*, 9, 2. Available: https://doi.org/10.17169/fqs-9.2.403 [Accessed 29/5/22].

O'Neill, M. & Harindranath, R. 2006. Theorising narratives of exile and belonging: the importance of biography and ethno-mimesis in "understanding" asylum. *Qualitative Sociology Review*, 2, 39–53.

Orange, D. M. 2017. *Climate Crisis, Psychoanalysis, and Radical Ethics*. New York: Routledge.

Ponton, L. 2019. Earthways: Environmental Arts Therapy for Repairing Insecure Attachment and Developing Creative Response-Ability in an Insecure World. *In:* Heginworth, I. S. & Nash, G. (eds.) *Environmental Arts Therapy: The Wild Frontiers of the Heart*. London: Routledge.

Potash, J. S. 2005. Rekindling the multicultural history of the American Art Therapy Association, Inc. *Art Therapy: Journal of the American Art Therapy Association*, 22, 184–188.

Randall, R. 2009. Loss and climate change: the cost of parallel narratives. *Eco-Psychology*, 1, 118–129.

Rust, M. 2020. *Towards an Ecopsychotherapy*. London: Confer Books.

Sajnani, N. & Kaplan, F. F. 2012. The creative arts therapies and social justice: a conversation between the editors of this special issue. *The Arts in Psychotherapy*, 39, 165–167.

Sharp, V. & Hickman, C. 2019. Eco-anxiety, eco-despair, eco-depression, eco-grief? Or maybe … eco-empathy? *Climate Crisis Conversations* [Podcast]. 13/10/19. Available: https://www.climatepsychologyalliance.org/~cpa/podcasts/402-podcast-eco-anxiety-eco-despair-eco-depression-eco-grief-or-maybe-eco-empathy [Accessed 10/02/22].

Stepney, S. A. 2019. Visionary architects of color in art therapy: Georgette Powell, Cliff Joseph, Lucille Venture, and Charles Anderson. *Art Therapy*, 36, 115–121.

Strathern, M. 1980. No Nature, No Culture: The Hagen Case. *In:* Strathern, M. & Maccormack, C. (eds.) *Nature, Culture, and Gender*. Cambridge: Cambridge University Press.

Talwar, S. 2003. Deconstructing Kaplan's views on multiculturalism. *Art Therapy*, 21, 44–48.

Talwar, S. 2010. An intersectional framework for race, class, gender, and sexuality in art therapy. *Art Therapy*, 27, 11–17.

Talwar, S. 2015. *Culture, Diversity, and Identity: From Margins to Center*. Great Britain: Taylor & Francis, 100.

Talwar, S. 2019a. *Art Therapy for Social Justice: Radical Intersections*. New York: Routledge.

Talwar, S. 2019b. Critiquing Art Therapy: History, Science and Representation. *In:* Talwar, S. (ed.) *Art Therapy for Social Justice: Radical Intersections*. New York: Routledge.

Waller, D. 1991. *Becoming a Profession: The History of Art Therapy in Britain, 1940–82*. London: Routledge.

Wiles, R., Clark, A. & Prosser, J. 2011. Visual Research Ethics at the Crossroads. *The SAGE Handbook of Visual Research Methods*. London: SAGE Publications Ltd.

Wilkinson, I. 2004. *Suffering: A Sociological Introduction*. London: Polity Press.

Wood, S. 2020. Beyond Messiaen's birds: the post-verbal world of dementia. *Medical Humanities*, 46, 73–83.

3 Belonging, imagination, and modernity

Having presented how the theory and practice of art therapy relates to social action and social justice, ecological thinking within psychology and psychotherapy, and arts-based research methods, this chapter is concerned with three sets of ideas of that I have found useful in navigating the distinct forms of crises that form the focus of the later chapters of this book. Belonging and imagination are two sets of ideas that I have had the longest association with, where they have informed my understanding of asylum and migration, domestic violence and abuse, and climate crisis. This reflects the regular appearance of reference to both belonging and imagination in literature concerned with those topics, within arts-based research texts, and ethnographic and sociological theory. Ideas associated with the study of modernity are a more recent component of my thinking about the topics and the method of enquiry, and gaining a more nuanced understanding of modernity has been the most important point of learning for me leading up to the development of this book and during its writing – especially, the acceptance of it being beyond redemption. Modernity is not normally an explicit topic of consideration within art therapy texts. Whilst I have shown in Chapter 2 how social action and social justice approaches to art therapy employ criticisms of contemporary social structures and contemporary economic models, whilst also drawing attention to the way in which a social change model is willing to address how the adoption of epistemologies operate within art therapy, modernity – as a historically situated confluence of believes and practices – mostly remains invisible within art therapy texts and therefore goes unexamined. Why is it important then to introduce the topic of modernity into art therapy thought and practice? My contention is that if modernity is the fundamental bedrock upon which contemporary western societies are founded then the fault lines and contradictions within modernity will be reflected in the practices that emerges from those societies. Art therapy is one of those practices. My second contention is that art therapy also contains within it the possibility of exposing those fault lines and contradictions, whilst offering up a different way of understanding many diverse worlds,

DOI: 10.4324/9781003142560-3

because it can bring to the surface, and embrace, what modernity masks and represses – as well as offering one way of imagining alternatives to modernity. And just as art therapy benefits from coming to terms with the revised understandings of ecology, nature, and politics that global heating has brought about, so too does it gain from a clearer appreciation of how modernity shapes and frames each of those understandings.

Belonging

In a comprehensive review of how belonging is conceived in contemporary sociological and political practice, Nira Yuval-Davis (2011) starts by stating that belonging is an emotional attachment to a feeling of being at home and of being safe, both in the present and in the hoped for future. Yuval-Davis also observes that home 'does not just generate positive and warm feelings. It also allows the safety as well as the emotional engagement to be, at times, angry, resentful, ashamed, indignant' (p. 10). Yuval-Davis argues that belonging is a foundational ingredient of both sociology and psychology. These are helpful starting points for framing what belonging means in the context that I am using it. From a psychological perspective, attachment theory is one that is very much focused upon early experiences of physical and emotional belonging that appears between parent and infant, whilst within Maslow's hierarchy of needs, belonging, alongside love, is placed midway between the foundation of physiological needs and the peak of self-actualisation (Maslow, 1987). The need for belongingness within Maslow's model includes being accepted, giving and receiving love, and connection to others. The history of sociology shows that 'many writings have been focused on the differential ways people belong to collectivities and states – as well as the social, economic, and political effects of instances of displacement of such belonging/s as a result of industrialization and/or migration' (Yuval-Davis, 2011, p. 11). The observed focus on how belonging has become a vital way of thinking about experiences of migration, asylum, and refuge, resonates with my own encounter with belonging as an important sociological concept that can complement theories of identity. For example, Maggie O'Neill frames belonging as an aspect of migration that a biographical approach to research can make use of with an eye towards producing knowledge that enhances social justice (O'Neill and Harindranath, 2006). Social justice, in this case, being concerned with the achievement of participatory democracy through enhancing the visibility of asylum seekers and their lived experiences that are more normally marginalised and hidden. Belonging within the context of the experiences of asylum and migration is part of a process that includes experiences of exile, displacement, transition, arrival, settlement, and the formation of transnational identities (O'Neill, 2008). It is related to the creation of home and the creation of safety. What also emerges as important for the creation of a sense of belonging for those seeking asylum is the role of community and of geographical place. In the context of art therapy, the value of O'Neill's focus upon belonging within experiences of migration and asylum is the use of the artistic and sensory expressions to enable the revealing and formation of narratives, stories and biographies. Within Chapter 4, I will expand upon how this arts-based and sense-based process operated in practice with, but here it is worth noting here that walking, poetry, map-making, painting, sculpture, video, and photography all appear as ways for participants, researchers, and artists, to work together and generate knowledge. About this method, O'Neill (2008) writes that 'the transformative role of this interdisciplinary undertaking involved the production of dialectical images emerging from biographical work dealing with lived experiences through working across the borders of art/ethnography in a collaborative process between participants' (no page). It is from this potential space, which an arts-based and sense-based methodology opens up, that a fuller understanding of belonging emerges for the purposes of the topics explored here. This is especially so where belonging is framed as a fluid, performative, and relational process that changes with time, place and as the constituents of communities, groups, and families change. In that framing, belonging is a process of becoming that emerges out of the dialogue between individuals and collectives (Yuval-Davis, 2011). Writing about the dialogue that exists between the individual and society, Yuval-Davis (2011), observes that identity 'is not individual or collective, but involves both, in an in-between perpetual state of "becoming," in which processes of identity construction, authorization and contestation take place' (p. 16). The sense that belonging is a dynamic process that exists between self and other also gives belonging an intersubjective quality in which there 'exists a constant and complex loop between individual (inter)action and social change, both affecting each other' (May, 2011, p. 367). The dynamic and intersubjective processes of belonging are to be found within the emotional and prosaic elements of everyday life. This can be seen in O'Neill's work, where belonging is additionally framed as being a process that is strongly manifested in embodied ways. O'Neill (2008) writes that '[t]he texts, objects and images emerging from this work have the potential to enable us to experience, imagine the overlapping spaces and places of exile, both physical, mental and social – the embodied experience of exile, displacement and emplacement/belonging' (no page). O'Neill is here referencing the experiences of exile, arrival, and settlement within asylum and migration, and of how art enables an imaginative dialogue to appear within the emplaced and embodied nature of that journey. The use of arts to access the embodied and sensual aspects of belonging is part of a wider movement within sociological and ethnographic research to incorporate different epistemologies

(Pink, 2007; Pink, 2009; Barone and Eisner, 2012) the scope of which was outlined in Chapter 2 when considering arts-based research and its relationship to new paradigm research.

What O'Neill refers to as a sense of belonging is a coalescence of the physical, emotional, relational, and political, and finds resonance in sociologist Vanessa May's use of belonging to understand the link between the everyday lives of individuals and social structures. May argues that belonging brings a unique understanding of the link between the individual self and the collective. May argues that dominant sociological models view modernity as leading to social and psychic fragmentation, at the same time as modernity increases the reflexive capacity of individuals as they try to respond to that very same fragmentation of common social bonds. Those models are founded on a romanticised and unsubstantiated view of past societies being fixed entities, with rigid sets of traditions and hierarchies, in contrast to modern societies that are in a constant state of flux and revolution. Those models also view large-scale social structures as being distinct from personal and everyday life. May (2011) contests these views, noting that 'traditions have not disappeared, but rather remain important features of contemporary societies though their nature and role may have shifted' (p. 365). Moreover, May proposes that the social and the personal are contingent upon each other, without a clear boundary between them. May puts forwards four reasons for why belonging can be considered as being an appropriate lens through which to view the relationship between self and society, writing: 'First, it is person-centred; second, it takes us into the everyday where the official and unofficial spheres interact; third, it allows us to view the relationship between self and society as complex; and fourth, its dynamic nature allows us to examine social change' (p. 364). Adopting a phenomenological position, May (2013) writes that 'a relational view of society entails that society is not a 'thing' that exists in and of itself, but is constantly in the making in the interactions between people' (p. 56); adding that 'society is constituted not only of how people relate to each other, but also their relationship to their material environment' (p. 57). As with the other understandings of belonging presented here, May places dynamism very centrally into the concept of belonging, so that belonging is seen to be a process of becoming, as much as it is a fixed state. Belonging is not a homogenous state in which all people of say a given nation or religion think about and experience their sense belonging in the same way. Belonging, for May, is also tied very firmly to the physicality of everyday life.

The distinction is made by May between belonging as something that comes about as individuals internalise shared experiences and condition, and belonging as something that is created in an intersubjective, collective, and politicised way. That later creation of belonging is subject to processes of discrimination, so that it becomes culturally and politically legitimate to ask who belongs and who does not belong to a given place? A relevant example of this being how psychotherapist and ethnographer Beth Collier (2021) observes that the British countryside is frequently experienced by people of colour as somewhere that they do not belong, noting that whilst there is a strong emotional connection with nature this is often rendered unsafe due to racist attitudes about who belongs in nature. Collier's work both highlights this experience and seeks to address it through leading programmes of nature-based practices for urban communities. At the same time, the progress made in the United Kingdom by *English Heritage* and the *National Trust* towards drawing attention to the links between the properties and estates in their care and British colonial history are critiqued for being unpatriotic and revisionist (Barker and Foster, 2021). Belonging frequently then becomes a political project, within which particular aspects of belonging are co-opted into the formation of political stories and myths. What is more, the politics of belonging is a process that takes on particular significance during times of crisis and tension; during war time or when there are heightened anxieties about terrorism for example (Yuval-Davis, 2011). Such crises expose the creative and conflictual tensions that appear between local, national, and international aspects of belonging that contemporary globalisation has brought about. It is helpful to think about belonging being intersectional in the same way that it is helpful to think about identity and participation in social life as being intersectional. An intersectional approach to belonging leads to a way of thinking about self as embedded and embodied within an intersection of relationships, places and times in which race, class, gender, sexuality, and disability contribute. As Eli Clare (2009) responds, when asked what their writing of location, disability, and sexuality is about: 'Inevitably, I answer, "Home". I mean place, body, identity, community, family as home' (p. xxv). As I will show in the following chapters, this point is important when considering belonging as a way of considering asylum and migration, or when considering global warming.

When placing belonging within an understanding of how art therapy can work with the types of crisis addressed here, it is necessary to also consider how a sense of *not* belonging appears, and in turn how the metaphor of bridging might be a useful way of addressing the gaps that appear between belonging and not belonging (Powell, 2017). Not only is bridging a useful concept for addressing how to reach across political divides, but also for exploring differences in heritage, culture, and religion. Those, and many other differences, are frequently employed as justifications for othering, whereby people are not given their full humanity. A process that for Powell occurs at an individual and a structural level. Othering is especially prevalent at this present time within much of the political discourse taking place within the United States and the United Kingdom, where a very distinct separation has appeared between different political and ideological positions, which was previously masked and managed by more centrist politicians and policies. Online platforms, or rather their algorithms and methods of encouraging engagement, have acted as accelerants for this separation, and provide limited scope for measured dialogue. Othering has become a normal component of online discourse, which in turn shapes broader political actions. At a more prosaic and visceral level, flooding in the UK town where I live in November 2019 made actual bridges across rivers unpassable for a short while (see Figure 3.1). This seemed like a pertinent visual metaphor for how to work across the differences I was encountering in my involvement with attempts to address climate change at that local level. I have come to think of bridging as a way in

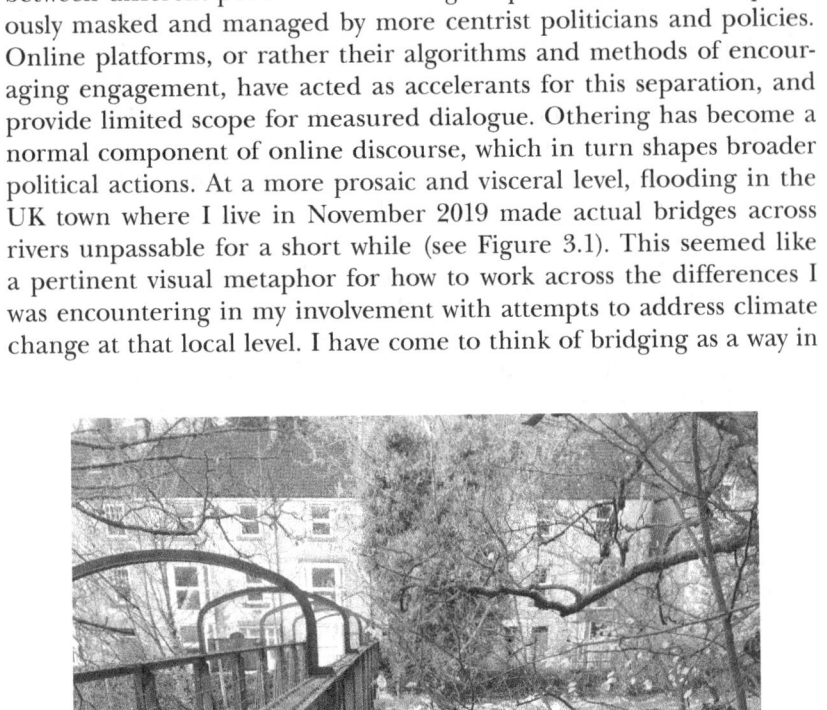

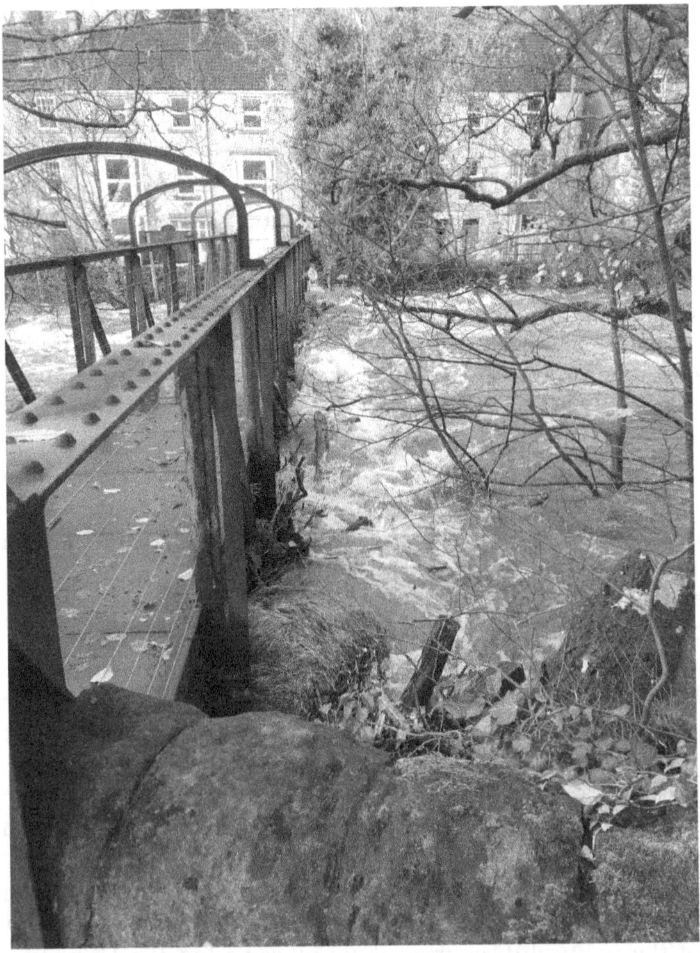

Figure 3.1 River Derwent flooding, November 2019 (Photo by Jamie Bird)

which to form and strengthen connections between people, to build a resilient community across rising, turbulent waters, where environmental and social justice is addressed equally. Again, for Powell (2017), bridging involves acknowledging the humanity in others, even when disagreements are strong. From my position, that acceptance of difference and humanity within bridging suggests how, when working together, we might learn to be with crisis and with trauma.

The most salient qualities of belonging, as I have presented them here, for my own practice and the arguments put forwards, are that belonging, with its attention to place, embodiment, and story, provides a dynamic up approach to conceiving of the relationship between the individual and the collective in a way that makes it very amenable to investigation through the use of arts-based research methods. Belonging closes the perceptual gaps between people, places, and social structures. It highlights that '[w]e do not merely spectate a society or participate in it. We are in it, we are it' (May, 2011, p. 375). Moreover, this is a position that has strong parallels to the focus upon the closing of the perceptual gap between the human and the other-than-human within ecological thought. Because of the role of place, physicality, time, and story, in how belonging is understood, it is amenable to being researched from an arts-based perspective because those same qualities are fundamental to the arts. And fundamental to that use of the arts as a research method, is how imagination is taken as a valid and effective way of generating knowledge.

Imagination

Imagination plays a central role within how I have used art therapy and arts-based research to address social action and justice. Imagination represents an epistemological approach that takes into account both the physical and political elements of the construction of knowledge. A feminist understanding of imagination emerges as a helpful way of drawing together those elements. As touched upon above, intersectionality appears within the construction of a fully worked out conception of belonging, where intersectionality is regarded as complementary to feminist-standpoint theory, which itself posits that it is essential to understand how any social agent is situated and positioned within social and political structures when approaching them (Yuval-Davis, 2011). Within this understanding of intersectionality, and of feminist-standpoint theory, reference is made to the role of situated knowledge and situated imagination within the construction of knowledge, where how knowledge and imagination appear are contingent upon intersecting features of disability, class, race, gender, sexuality, geography, and so forth, as well as the intersecting appearance of thought, feeling and sensation. These are important epistemological positions that exist in parallel to positivistic ways of knowing and so are worth paying further attention to.

A starting point to thinking about imagination and expanding on those points above is to take quotations from two authors that I have called upon already, and to think through the implications of their claims. The first is from Norman Denzin (2000), who, when considering the potential of new paradigm qualitative research texts, states that '[t]he moral text is utopian. It imagines how the world could be different' (p. 261). Denzin repeats this assertion when claiming that the value of any piece of new paradigm research can be judged to be worthy of the title when it can be shown that '[i]t will criticize how things are and will imagine how they could be different' (p. 262). The second quotation comes from the writing of philosopher Sandra Harding. Writing about feminist-standpoint theory, Harding (1998) provides a critique of a number of feminist epistemologies, suggesting that 'different epistemologies offer possibilities for different distributions of political power' (p. 175) in terms of how they legitimise different kinds of knowledge. For example, when considering the limits of empiricism, Harding claims that it overvalues objective reason whilst undervaluing subjective, emotional, and embodied knowledge. In contrast, a feminist-standpoint epistemology is one that positions women's lived experience at the centre of the generation of knowledge and action. It is because of this centring of lived experience that feminist-standpoint theory argues for the importance within critical enquiry of starting off thought from the lives of others. For Harding, '[s]tarting off research from women's lives will generate less partial and distorted accounts not only of women's lives but also of men's lives and of the whole social order' (Harding, 2004, p. 128). The inclusion of men's lives here recognises the social construction of gendered experience for both women and men, and by extension the social construction of other aspects of identity, and the necessity of acknowledging different positions in creating knowledge. I would argue that if feminist-standpoint epistemology is interested in generating knowledge that emerges from more than one position then it must also value different forms and expression of knowledge, including embodied experiences and imagination. Moreover, I suggest that it is this potential for the valuing of different forms of knowledge within feminist-standpoint theory, including imagination and embodied knowing, which creates a bridge to thinking about arts-based methodologies.

Writing with Marcel Stoetzler, Yuval-Davis provides a fuller examination of the place of imagination within feminist-standpoint theory (Stoetzler and Yuval-Davis, 2002), where they draw upon 17th-century European philosopher Baruch Spinoza's meditation on the relationship between the mind and the body. They identify that Spinoza 'conceives of the mind not as an entity distinct from and opposed to the body, but as the body's self-awareness' (p. 323). Within Spinoza's philosophy, imagination plays an important role in the mediation of senses to that self-awareness, and also acts as the link between the corporeal awareness of the individual and the awareness of other beings, whom together share the mental and physical space that forms his concept of community and political society. This attention to the notion of the relationship between body and mind confirms Leavy's (2007) suggestion concerning the challenge made by feminist thought upon mind-body dualism, and helps to consider how imagination and the body are related. The situated nature of Spinoza's understanding of imagination, in part because it is predicated upon corporeal bodies and personal habits, is highlighted by Stoetzler and Yuval-Davis (2002). In thinking about the implications of this upon feminist-standpoint theory, they state that 'the transformation of situated experience to situated knowledge, in particular, are impossible to understand without incorporating a notion of the situated imagination' (p. 325). A consideration of the situated nature of imagination is therefore central to Stoetzler and Yuval-Davis' understanding of imagination within feminist-standpoint theory.

The consideration of imagination being related to, and situated upon, the material and corporeal quality of the body brings to mind again Genevive Lloyd's exposure, in *The Man of Reason* (1993), of a tradition of gender bias that appears within conceptions of reason and rationality within western philosophy that runs from Plato through to Sartre and de Beauvoir. Reason, within that tradition, is shown by Lloyd to be variously related to concepts of nature: in opposition to it, complementing it, transcending it, emerging from it, and as observing and reflecting upon it. Lloyd argues that in these various understandings, nature is associated with the corporeal body, and by turns with the feminine, both as a metaphor, and as way of contrasting the public and transcendent qualities of reason with the private and personal qualities of the passions and feelings. In this way, the feminine becomes related to the passions, the emotions, and the corporeal; each of which is considered the enemy of reason. Nature, Lloyd argues, is represented as uncontrolled and wild, though open to being known and dominated, and by conjoining the feminine with the natural and the corporeal, whether through metaphor or through direct comparison, both nature and the feminine are equated with the non-rational and as the object of reason rather than its subject. In the hierarchy of epistemologies, reason, associated as it is with the masculine, comes to be seen as occupying a more privileged position than the passions or feelings that are equated with ideas of the feminine. This gendering of reason, despite the ideal of a transcendent neutrality claimed for reason, Lloyd argues, leads to a position whereby reason is valued above other forms of knowledge and contributes to women and men defining themselves and their experiences in a limited way 'to the disadvantage of women and men alike' (p. 108).

From this perspective, a truly gender-neutral conception of reason is a vision for the future rather than a present possibility. What a gender-neutral conception of reason might be like is not set out by Lloyd, although, like Stoetzler and Yuval-Davis (2002), there is a turn to Spinoza and his grounding of thought within the body to think through an alternative to bodiless reason, when it is stated that 'Spinoza opens up the possibility of taking seriously differences – grounded in body – in the context, style, motivation or interest of reasoning, without denying the commonalities that arise from the shared humanity of our differently sexed bodies' (Lloyd, 1993, p. xv). The situated and corporeal nature of mental processes, including reason, as conceived of by Spinoza, is presented then as a quality that is philosophically legitimate, rather than one to be transcended.

Of particular relevance to the discussion about imagination is the observation made by Lloyd about René Descartes' separation of the body and the mind; she writes that '[h]e saw the encroachments of non-intellectual passion, sense or imagination as coming not from lower parts or aspects of the soul, but from altogether outside the soul – as intrusions from the body' (Lloyd, 1993, p. 46). Following Lloyd's argument about gender and reason, it would seem then that if imagination is placed within the tradition of western philosophy as being counter to, and separate from reason, in the same way as the passions and the senses, because of its relation to the body, then by implication philosophical conceptions of imagination are gendered in the same way as reason. The separation of reason from imagination along the line of the body can be contrasted with Spinoza's concept of imagination that is explored later by Lloyd when writing with Moira Gatens (Gatens and Lloyd, 1999), and later still by Gatens alone who approaches Spinoza from a feminist perspective (Gatens, 2009). In those readings of Spinoza, it is argued that the corporeal quality of imagination is understood by Spinoza to be its defining feature, and that 'imagination involves awareness of other bodies at the same time as our own. Our bodies retain traces of the changes brought about in them by the impinging of other bodies' (Gatens and Lloyd, 1999, p. 23). From this perspective, the relationship between reason and imagination takes on a particular tone:

> The order of imagination is not the order of reason. But reason can come to an understanding of the associations which operate between images, of the ways in which they are affected by emotion, and of the ways in which those interactions of imagination and emotion are themselves affected by the collectivities into which human beings are drawn through interaction with bodies similar to their own.
>
> (p. 24)

Imagination then, within a Spinozian philosophy, becomes both a legitimate focus of rational inquiry as well as being itself a method of inquiry, rather than a phenomenon to be transcended, especially so where social and political relations between people are the area of concern. Reason and imagination thus become related through their shared attachment to the corporeal, with each being embedded within the intersubjectivity of social relations. In considering the place of reason and imagination within collective thought, Stoetzler and Yuval-Davis call attention to Cornelius Castoriadis' (1994, 1987 cited in Stoetzler and Yuval-Davis, 2002) concept of a 'socially constitutive imaginary' (p. 326), where it is proposed that societies are dictated less by rationality and reason, and more by imaginary concepts of themselves. In the same way, Gatens and Lloyd (1999) argue that in Spinoza's understanding, imagination 'becomes lodged in social practices and institutional structures in ways which make it an anonymous feature of collective mental life' (p. 39). The relationship between imagination and reason becomes one of coexistence, albeit one that is often below the surface of social or political consciousness. And where Murray Bookchin (2015) discerns that '[n]or can imagination be excluded from History, but it is an imagination that must be elucidated by reason' (p. 106), there is the recognition that both reason and imagination are needed in equal measure to create the kinds of political structures that social ecology requires to come into existence.

If reason and imagination are located within the situated and corporeal nature of human thought, it can be argued that a more radical version of the relationship between reason and imagination would be to say that they are of one and the same kind: that reason is the refinement of imagination, and a refinement that is achieved through methods of analysis and scrutiny. When it is taken that reason is tied to the body, it is no longer possible to appeal to a pre-existing transcendent and universal space where rational thought by itself can access truth; it is instead an embodied process that uses imagination to lead thought out of the immediate and the personal, into the shared social and political space of other imagining and reasoning bodies. Imagination, where it is related to, and emerges from the body, leads not only to the notion of situated imagination, as set forth by Stoetzler and Yuval-Davis (2002), but also, I suggest, to the idea of embodied imagination. In this understanding, embodiment and imagination thus become intimately related. Imagination becomes a legitimate form of understanding that is not separate from reason; rather they together constitute a process of thought that is embodied, situated, and dependent upon other thinking bodies. To which, we might want to add the inclusion of other-than-human bodies.

As well as considering the relationship between imagination and reason and their embodied social qualities, the relationship between imagination and time is of importance when considering social action and justice. Reviewing the historical appearance of imagination within western philosophy, Richard Kearney (1991) suggests that the 'imagined object may be a synthesis of past, present and future time' (p. 54). In this understanding, acts of imagination, when combined with rational analysis and projected forwards in time in the form of 'fantastic imaginings that change history' (Haraway, 1993 cited in Stoetzler and Yuval-Davis, 2002, p. 326), can become a way of considering and shaping the future. Such a claim for imagination fits with the aim of political change and emancipation that social action and social justice strives for, as well as aligning with the principles that underpin the feminist project of emancipation. This imagining of fair and just futures becomes a key objective of domestic violence and abuse research that is informed by feminism, which will become clearer in Chapter 4, as well as within the research of experiences such as migration and climate crisis that involve complex and uncertain trajectories.

When reviewing Spinoza's philosophy, Gatens and Lloyd (1999) observe that the 'bodily awareness of it's [the mind] nature involves awareness of the past as well as the present and inevitably gives rise to expectations of the contingent future' (p. 34). And whilst thinking in detail about gender and embodiment, Paula-Irene Villa (2011) writes that '[e]mbodiment is always fragile and transitory, never done' (p. 179), so that for Villa the embodiment of gender is not about being, but is instead a process of becoming. This suggests that the process of becoming is a complex ongoing story in which individuals perform personal interpretations of collective ideas about gender. In Villa's understanding of embodiment, people become both what they imagine is expected of them but also what they desire for themselves, with those imaginings and desires being informed by complex and dynamic intersectional forces in which embodiment is a 'social process, expanding over time and space' (p. 181). This expansion over time, following Spinoza's understanding of the corporeal nature of imagination, can be read as pointing towards a view of the future being contingent upon an embodied imagination that is capable of being expansive and dynamic. This is an important consideration where research or therapeutic interventions asks people to express their imagined futures in addition to their past and present lives.

The point made above by Villa about embodiment being fragile and transitory, resonates with Ann Murphy's (2012) observations about the place of vulnerability and ambiguity within feminist ontology and political imagination. Building upon Michéle Le Doeuff's (Le Doeuff, 2002) examination of the denial of imagination and imagery within philosophy, Murphy argues that it is vulnerability that makes us open to others, to their corporeal, ontological, and ethical otherness, which in turn has the potential to enable empathy. Conversely, Murphy argues that corporeal vulnerability can just as easily provoke a retreat from what is imagined to be the other in fear and repulsion. From this perspective, imagination, and its association to the vulnerable corporal body, becomes a potential source of wounding and violence as well as a prompt for caring and compassion. In Murphy's view, both vulnerability and imagination occupy ambiguous positions within philosophy – something to be drawn back from as well as something to be approached. Murphy talks of an 'emergent feminist ontology of corporeal vulnerability' (2012, p. 99) and considers the implications of an ethics based upon vulnerability, where the ambiguous nature of vulnerability is embraced rather than denied so that the beneficial components of care and compassion do not become 'concealed by [vulnerability's] overwhelming association with violence' (p. 98) that so much philosophy espouses. Murphy calls attention to the way in which images of violence permeate continental philosophy's accounts of identity and difference, and argues for a conception of self and otherness that is based upon an interdependence that is both ambiguous and vulnerable. As such, any idea of an emancipatory future is required to acknowledge and embrace the ambiguity that is inherent within corporeal vulnerability and its associated influence upon imagination (of self and of others), rather than attempt to transcend it. In Chapter 4, Murphy's conception of ambiguity and vulnerability, will emerge as a useful way of understanding how the women who took part in the work related to domestic abuse represented their memories and imaginations.

The implications for social action art therapy of paying attention to the features of imagination examined here are that it brings to the surface ways of knowing and being that complement what is cognitive and empirical. Art therapy has a natural affinity with imagination because of how it combines a sensitivity to creative processes, and in how it embraces those aspects of contemporary psychology and psychoanalysis that place an emphasis upon imagination as an important psychic process. Where there is an opportunity to expand this appreciation of imagination within art therapy, is in considering the place of imagination within political thought and action. A feminist understanding of imagination, along with an intersectional perspective upon social hierarchies, brings that political perspective to the surface, with the addition of a philosophy of embodiment grounding imagination within the everyday and the interpersonal.

Modernity

Alongside belonging and imagination being fundamental to how I make use of social action therapy is the development of a fuller understanding of the foundations of those social and political systems of thought and practice that create the contemporary world. That foundation is modernity. An important point to hold in mind about the anthropocene and climate crisis is that it is no accident of history. Christophe Bonneuil and Jean-Baptise Fressoz (2017) observe that both capitalism and modernity are frequently and naively blamed for the emergence of the Anthropocene, where we do not have a full historical picture of what deliberate and incremental decisions have been made about the use of natural resources. They provide examples of where solar and wind energy have been deployed widely and efficiently within recent US history, but have succumb to the political lobbying of nuclear, oil, and gas industries. Rather than all aspects of modernity being at fault, there is a particular form of capitalist modernity that leads to the inefficient use of finite natural resources being valued above efficiency if it leads to the accumulation of capital and power in the hands of a small number of people. Although appearing as a rather dispersed and abstract concept, modernity is a necessary area of attention because it encapsulates a set of belief systems and objectives that frame much of contemporary belief, thought, and action. Whilst the western world has been primarily shaped by modernity over the last four centuries, the processes of colonialism and globalisation has seen it attaining dominance as a way of thinking and acting in most other parts of the world. Given the difficulty of imagining and operating outside of modernity, it is relevant to ask: *What features of modernity need to be brought forwards for consideration at this point that has relevance to social action art therapy and working with crisis?* Modernity is a vast subject area, and one that ostensibly dictates the structure of thought within contemporary society. Thinking from a position outside of modernity presents challenges to what is considered valid, because of it how it has become *the* dominant political and cultural ideology. And, whereas a critique of modernity and of capitalism appears within the framing of art therapy as an aid to social justice (Talwar, 2019), and within nature-based expressive therapies (Atkins & Snyder, 2018), neither are explicitly addressed within social action art therapy literature. A clearer understanding of modernity will be needed therefore, even if a complete view is not possible from the privileged and secure position that I occupy within modernity.

Two analyses of modernity are of particular relevance to social action therapy. The first analysis is presented by French sociologist Bruno Latour. The second by Ecuadorian philosopher Bolivar Echeverría. Latour's analysis of modernity is relevant because of his extensive interrogation of its role within the formation of, and response to, ecological crises; whilst Echeverría's analysis is relevant because of the relationship he identifies between modernity, capitalism, colonialism, and racism. In Latour's reading (1993), the genesis of modernity is located in the twin projects of political emancipation as outlined in Thomas Hobbes' *Leviathan*, and the establishment of experimental science via Robert Boyle's construction of, and experimentation with, artificial vacuums. Contemporaries, working and writing in the 17th century in the chaotic wake of the English civil war, Hobbes and Boyle both set out, within politics and the natural sciences respectively, to challenge those received traditions of thought and behaviour that dominated before that point. Latour argues that there is within modernity a duel objective of domination and emancipation, which is driven by a perpetual desire for progress and revolution, observing that '[t]he adjective "modern" designates a new regime, an acceleration, a rupture, a revolution in time. When the word "modern"," "modernization"," or "modernity" appears, we are defining, by contrast, an archaic and stable past' (p. 10). Because modernity creates a state of perpetual revolution in its seeking out of constant progress, so too does it create a sense of perpetual crisis. There is a divide within modernity that takes place between other-than-human nature, and human culture, and there are fundamental contradictions in how they are conceived as both transcendent and immanent. Nature is conceptualised as not our construction; but its laws are artificially constructed within the laboratory. Society is conceptualised as our own free construction; whilst also being constrained by natural forces that are beyond our will. From these contradictions, a constitution emerges, with three associated guarantees. Latour articulates this constitution and the three guarantees in the following way:

> First guarantee: even though we construct Nature, Nature is as if we did not construct it. Second guarantee: even though we do not construct Society, Society is as if we did construct it. Third guarantee: Nature and Society must remain absolutely distinct: the work of purification must remain absolutely distinct from the work of mediation.
>
> (p. 32)

Whilst human culture and other-than-human nature are made distinct and purified within their isolated vacuums, the continuation of their intermingling is mediated and then relegated to what Latour refers to as hybrids, writing that '[t]he essential point of this modern Constitution is that it renders the work of mediation that assembles hybrids invisible, unthinkable, unrepresentable' (p. 34). The web of delicate and subtle interactions between objects, places, actions, and beliefs, within a pre-modern understanding of destiny and causality is replaced by a demonstration of cause and effect between tightly controlled variables, witnessed and theorised by invisible and neutralised human observers. Hybrids are ways of making sense in an everyday way of the invisible complexity that purification and specialisation creates. For example, how can we mentally hold together simultaneously, something as opaque as theoretical physics alongside the obtuse workings of monetary debt markets, or the terrible scale of hunger and poverty in the world? Latour therefore asks not if we are still modern, but, have we ever been modern? The answer for Latour is no, we have never been modern, because we have to operate both within the constitutional purification of nature and society and the guarantees of modernity, at the same time as taking account of the proliferation of hybrids. It is, for Latour, when we are holding these positions simultaneously that we are being non-modern.

It is where hybrids are suppressed that processes of translation and mediation are required to make those hybrids both expressible and knowable. Referencing Dona Haraway (Haraway, 1991), Latour suggests that we need to slow down the proliferation of monsters and tricksters; that we must work to make those monsters legitimate. Naming monsters and tricksters, Latour is referring to those hybrid explanations and translations that implicitly lie beneath the surface of separation and purification of other-than-human nature from human culture that modernity explicitly enacts. Bruno Latour's thesis is that where a non-modern anthropological approach to contemporary western society is applied, naturalised phenomena as studied by the natural sciences, social process of power and hierarchy as studied by social and political sciences, and the forms and content of cultural discourse, are not examined as separate entities. Rather than being separated out as if they existed in their own individual, artificial vacuums, they are instead allowed to come together, and their continued coexistence brought to the surface. An expression of this process, in the context of the Covid-19 global pandemic is teacher and writer Bayo Akomolafe's (2020) reference to Èṣù, the Yoruba, West Africa, version of the trickster character that appears at times of transition and crisis: 'In a sense, viruses behave like tricksters. Like Èṣù, the devious Yoruba god of the "Orita" (poorly translated as crossroads but more poetically understood as the monstrous place where the three ways cut through each other), viruses in their transversal showing-up as extra-modern entities are investigators of difference, composers of multiplicity' (p. 17). The significance of this set of ideas about hybrids and monsters, for art therapy, is in how their proliferation beneath the surface of society, aligns with art therapy's knowledge of and comfort with images from the individual and collective unconscious. Art therapy, although prone to a process of division and purification where it places psychological understandings foremost (which it cannot but fail to do, being situated within modernity), is very capable of taking account of hybrid images, objects, and stories. What is more, I would argue that a social action approach to art therapy, in its attempts to draw together psychological and sociological perspectives, makes hybrid images and objects more explicit.

Where Latour suggests that we have never been truly modern, Echeverría suggests that we are not modern enough because the future imagined by modernity, and the present created by capitalism, are incompatible with each other. Modernity offers the promise of a society of post-scarcity and emancipation achieved through the technological manipulation and coordination of nature and society, whereas capitalism creates scarcity and inequality in the pursuit of excess profits through the exploitation of resources and labour and the construction of demand driven markets (Echeverría, 2019). According to Echeverría, we (those of us born into or educated into western or global north states) can be considered to be not modern enough because we hold on to the historical memory of absolute resource scarcity, along with the stories, myths, and methods of social management that the long memory of that scarcity has created within human history. For Echeverría, that memory of how to manage absolute scarcity can be traced back to the birth of agriculture – an observation also made by Timothy Morton (Morton, 2016), but with the twist of highlighting the romanticism inherent in trying to imagine pre-agricultural society from afar. Despite the capacity and potential for the technological components of modernity to adequately supply the needs of all people within the constraints set by the other-than-human world, and ethnographic and archaeological examples of societies consciously choosing to manage scarcity in many different ways (Graeber and Wengrow, 2021), a capitalist version of modernity requires the artificial reconstruction of partial and absolute scarcity in order to create debt, capital, and speculation. The observation made by Echeverría (2019) that modernity, where it fails to fulfil the objective of the human and the other-than-human working in harmony, 'cannot yet fully affirm itself over its own basis instead of continuing to sustain itself on the archaic, Neolithic technique based upon the conquest of nature' (p. 13) repeats the proposition that we are – as yet – not modern enough.

Further to the continued creation of scarcity, Echeverría contends that the capitalist version of modernity also requires the creation of atomised individuals who can internalise and perform 'whiteness.' Echeverria uses quotation marks in this way to represent how 'whiteness' is socially constructed and open to deconstruction, and to differentiate performed 'whiteness' from ethnic whiteness. Essential aspects of 'whiteness,' as Echeverría sees it appearing within capitalist modernity, involves the making of personal sacrifices in order to service the market place of production and consumption, and the valuing of the protestant and puritan ethics and modes of behaviour above all other ethical codes or other indigenous versions of morality, or other possible versions of modernity. Echeverría (2019) discerns that:

> being authentically modern came to include among its essential conditions belonging in some way or to some extent to the white race, and consequently also to relegating, as a matter of principle,

all singular or collective individuals that were 'of colour' or simply foreign, or 'non-Western' to the abstract field of the pre-, anti-, or non-modern (or non-human).

(p. 41)

For Echeverría, it is the valuing of 'whiteness' over other versions of being human that enables and accelerates racism and white supremacy within capitalist modernity. Violence appears within capitalist modernity in the form of the creation of, and the separation of 'whiteness,' from other versions of being human – '[t]hus the "original sin" of all liberal societies is that they are wrought through violence and depend upon an ongoing process of coercion' (Kish and Quilley, 2017, p. 310). As an alternative version of modernity, observing responses to capitalist modernity within Mexico, Echeverría implies that there is a desire and a need to imagine versions of modernity that are neither wedded to capitalism or to 'whiteness.' Echeverría indicates that this might appear in the form of a baroque version of modernity: a version of modernity that is theatrical, poetic, and pluralistic, and one that embraces and makes visible those contradictions that are set up between nature and culture. And perhaps a version of modernity where the original principle of emancipation is extended to include that which is other-than-human.

Summary

For the purposes of thinking about art therapy and its connection to social action, belonging, imagination, and modernity offer ways of considering the relationship between singular individuals and the social contexts that they find themselves situated in. Belonging, and not-belonging, has been presented here as a sense of being part of – or excluded from – community and place, with attention drawn to the physical qualities and manifestations of belonging. Imagination, in a similar way, is framed as an epistemology that is contingent upon body, place, and time. As such, an analysis has been presented whereby both belonging and imagination are considered to be situated within, and therefore contingent upon and shaped by social contexts. This sets up a state of tension when the dominant version of modernity places individuals and bodies of knowledge within their own isolated and atomised vacuums, at the same time as creating a hierarchy of people and knowledge that is kept in place through violence. The tension created by that difference reappears within those hybrid objects (thoughts, feelings, actions, dreams, and physical things) that act as mediators and translators for the complexity and difference that modernity seeks to suppress. Social action art therapy is one way of bringing those hybrids to the surface in a way that allows their existence and knowledge to be appreciated and acted upon consciously. The suggestion is made that there are other ways of being modern – even of being other-than-modern – of imagining and finding alternatives to capitalist modernity that can take account of historical and ongoing diversity within how societies structure themselves. That there might more than one way of imagining what it means to belong. Chapters 4 and 5 will make manifest the ideas that have been presented in this and Chapter 3 in the context of working to understand and respond to migration and asylum, domestic violence and abuse, and climate crisis.

References

Akomolafe, B. 2020. *I, Coronavirus. Mother. Monster. Activist.* [Online]. Available: https://bayoakomolafe.net/project/i-coronavirus-mother-monster-activist/ [Accessed 31/12/20].

Barker, A. & Foster, P. 2021. The 'war on woke': who should shape Britain's history? *Financial Times*, 11/6/21.

Barone, T. & Eisner, E. W. 2012. *Arts Based Research*. London: Sage.

Bonneuil, C. & Fressoz, J.-B. 2017. *The Shock of the Anthropocene: The Earth, History, and Us*. London: Verso Books.

Bookchin, M. 2015. *The Next Revolution: Popular Assemblies* and the *Promise* of *Direct Democracy*. London: Verso Books.

Clare, E. 2009. *Exile and Pride: Disability, Queeness, and Liberation*. Durham, NC: Duke University Press.

Collier, B. 2021. *Nature connectors* [Online]. Available: https://wildinthecity.org.uk/nature-connectorsprogramme/ [Accessed 20/01/21].

Denzin, N. K. 2000. Aesthetics and the Practices of Qualitative Inquiry. *Qualitative Inquiry*, 6, 256–265.

Echeverría, B. 2019. *Modernity and "Whiteness"*. Cambridge: Polity Press.

Gatens, M. (ed.) 2009. *Feminist Interpretations of Benedict Spinoza*. Pennsylvania: Pennsylvania State University Press.

Gatens, M. & Lloyd, G. 1999. *Collective Imaginings: Spinoza, Past and Present*. London: Routledge.

Graeber, D. & Wengrow, D. 2021. *The Dawn of Everything: A New History of Humanity*. London: Penguin.

Haraway, D. 1991. *Simians, Cyborgs, and Women: The Reinvention of Nature*. New York: Chapman & Hall.

Harding, S. 1998. Can Men Be Subjects of Feminist Thought? *In:* Digby, T. (ed.) *Men Doing Feminism*. London: Routledge.

Harding, S. 2004. *The Feminist Standpoint Theory Reader: Intellectual & Political Controversies*. London: Routledge.

Kearney, R. 1991. *Poetics of Imagination: From Husserl to Lyotard*. London: Harper Collins.

Kish, K. & Quilley, S. 2017. Wicked dilemmas of scale and complexity in the politics of degrowth. Ecological Economics, 142, 306–317.

Latour, B. 1993. *We Have Never Been Modern*. New York: Harvester Wheatsheaf.

Leavy, P. 2007. *Merging Feminist Principles and Art-Based Methodologies* American Sociological Association Annual Conference, New York. https://www.asanet.org/sites/default/files/2007_annual_meeting_program.pdf (accessed 23/6/22).

Le Doeuff, M. 2002. *The Philosophical Imaginary*. London: Columbia University Press.

Lloyd, G. 1993. *The Man of Reason; 'Male' & 'Female' in Western Philosophy* (2nd ed.). Routledge.

Maslow, A. H. 1987. *Motivation and Personality*. Delhi, India: Pearson Education.

May, V. 2011. Self, belonging and social change. *Sociology*, 45, 363–378.

May, V. 2013. *Connecting Self to Society: Belonging in a Changing World*. Basingstoke: Palgrave.

Morton, T. 2016. *Dark Ecology: For a Logic of Future Coexistence*. New York: Columbia University Press.

Murphy, A. 2012. *Violence and the Philosophical Imaginary*. New York: State University of New York Press.

O'Neill, M. 2008. Transnational refugees: the transformative role of art? *Forum Qualitative Sozialforschung/Forum: Qualitative Social Research*, 9, 2. Available: https://doi.org/10.17169/fqs-9.2.403 [Accessed 29/5/22].

O'Neill, M. & Harindranath, R. 2006. Theorising narratives of exile and belonging: the importance of biography and ethno-mimesis in "understanding" asylum. *Qualitative Sociology Review*, 2, 39–53.

Pink, S. 2007. *Doing Visual Ethnography*. London: Sage.

Pink, S. 2009. *Doing Sensory Ethnography*. London: Sage.

Powell, J. A. 2017. *John A. Powell on How Bridging Creates Conditions to Solve Problems* [Online]. Berkeley: Othering and Belonging Institute. Available: https://belonging.berkeley.edu/john-powell-how-bridging-creates-conditions-solve-problems [Accessed 26/01/21].

Stoetzler, M. & Yuval-Davis, N. 2002. Standpoint theory, situated knowledge and the situated imagination. *Feminist Theory*, 3, 315–33.

Talwar, S. 2019. *Art therapy for social justice: radical intersections*. New York: Routledge.

Villa, P. 2011. Embodiment Is Always More: Intersectionality, Subjection and the Body. *In:* Lutz, H., Vivar, M. & Supik, L. (eds.) *Framing Intersectionality: Debates on a Multi-Faceted Concept in Gender Studies*. Farnham: Ashgate Publishing Limited.

Yuval-Davis, N. 2011. *The Politics of Belonging: Intersectional Contestations*. London: Sage.

4 Violence, asylum, and refuge

This chapter explores how experiences of violence, asylum, and refuge can be viewed as examples of the fractured nature of modernity that was put forward in Chapter 3, and of how they disrupt belonging and produce trauma. I will provide examples of how the arts can contribute to bringing to light and better understanding what such experiences look and feel like. I make reference to my involvement in the *Sense of Belonging* research project and associated exhibition, which was led by Professor Maggie O'Neill (O'Neill, 2009). I also refer to the *Artrefuge* art therapy initiative led by art therapist Bobby Lloyd at the Calais refugee camps. A substantial part of this chapter will explore the arts-based research that I have conducted, exploring how women who have experienced domestic violence and abuse tell their stories. The idea of a transitional story is the key theme to emerge from that work and to be carried forward in responding to the climate crisis. It is argued that the arts – in the form of therapy and research – can contribute to the formation of transitional stories, in which resistance, adaptation, and a remade sense of self and belonging can emerge. I define a transitional story as one that entails the representation of physical and emotional movement between places, movement through time, and changes in familial and social relationships. In the context of the work done with women who have experienced domestic violence and abuse, together these transitions contribute to the changing ways in which women perceive themselves and engage in acts of agency and resistance as they rebuild their sense of self and belonging. There are elements of these stories that contain acts of action and of control, and elements that highlight barriers to the achievement of goals and desired outcomes. A transitional story is one that encompasses the past, the present, and the future, and one that encourages imaginative movements back and forth between points in time in a non-linear fashion.

Having devoted considerable time to setting out a theory of social action art therapy in previous chapters – one that references social justice movements, ecotherapies, and arts-based research, incorporates the concepts of belonging and imagination, whilst also being offered

DOI: 10.4324/9781003142560-4

as a method of rethinking modernity – this chapter provides content that is applied to particular contexts and experiences. Rather, this chapter provides a context within which the many ideas introduced so far come into contact with lived experiences. Two sets of experiences are considered: asylum and refuge as they appear within migration between countries, and asylum and refuge as they appear within experiences of domestic violence and abuse. Both sets of experiences involve encounters with violence, both involve disruption to the social self, and both change how the past and the future is imagined and narrated. Both entail the formation of transitional stories. Through considering how art therapy and arts-based research has been used to both address and better understand migration and domestic abuse, in my own work and that of others, an applied sense of social action art therapy will emerge. Furthermore, by paying attention to how the arts can address the shared features of asylum, migration, and of domestic violence and abuse, the scene is set for exploring how social action art therapy can address the effects of climate crisis, which is itself also an experience of violence and disruption. Before presenting those examples, I first will put forward an understanding of violence that helps to think about the forms of crisis focused on here. This includes an appreciation of violence as it unfolds slowly, and the effects of violence upon the idea of self.

The chapter includes visual images that act as examples of transitional stories, the importance of physical spaces and objects within the remaking of the self, how relationships contribute to belonging, and the role of memory and imagination in shaping ideas about the future. These visual examples include images made by research participants, and who gave consent for their images and words produced in the original research to be disseminated appropriately.

Slow violence and the remaking of the self

Continuing to pay attention to modernity, the fundamental role of violence within the maintenance of globalised capitalism and the nation state is expressed by Vanessa Andreotti in her critical approach to the teaching of global citizenship and international development. Andreotti writes that '[a]t the ontological layer of critique, there is a notion that the problems plaguing the system are in fact of its own making, and further, that the system has always been subsidized by the violence of exploitation, ecocide, and genocide' (Andreotti et al., 2018, p. 28). The system referred to being the various institutions and structures that go to form an interconnected global economy and set of political positions – what Andreotti refers to as 'the house that modernity built' (Andreotti et al., 2015; Andreotti et al., 2018). In order to remain standing, the house of modernity requires the denigration of people and ideas that are deemed to be deviant, dangerous, or not worthy of truly belonging inside the house of modernity. It also requires the stratification and division of the interior floors and rooms of the house, so as to maintain a hierarchy of privilege, power, and wealth. Important to this understanding of modernity is the recognition that rather than the denigrated being excluded from modernity entirely, they are instead assigned to the margins of modernity, and exploited, primarily through exploitative labour. This marginalisation and exploitation operates within and across national borders. Denigration and division, where they cannot be achieved through the management of consent within the classroom or the media, are achieved by acts of actual physical harm. That violence has in turn made the very thing it seeks to protect vulnerable to collapse, so the house of modernity is now a fragile dwelling, in which multiple points of stress conspire towards its collapse. The fragile house, as a metaphor for the state of modernity in the 21st century, is pertinent to the concern for belonging and home when contemplating responses to asylum, domestic violence and abuse, and global heating. It both illustrates and reflects how a place of safety for one group can become a place of fear and non-safety for other groups. The appearance of a place that is unsafe for many groups can be observed in the government-sanctioned creation and maintenance of what is termed a 'hostile environment' within the United Kingdom; that whilst originally aimed at supressing migration into the United Kingdom, reflects a broader attitude and set of official sanctions towards those who are already vulnerable due to economic or health reasons. Similarly, the concept of solastalgia (Albrecht, 2005) can be viewed as the psychological and cultural expression of the emotional cost of modernity's fragility, where there is a mourning both for the actual and the feared loss of place as a consequence of economic growth and development, and the subsequent violence enacted upon the land. Once safe places now become unsafe. Places of refuge become places of danger and risk.

In this conception of modernity then, violence occupies a central place and sets the context within which more specific expressions of violence appear. And violence, in its various physical, emotional and coercive forms, has an obvious role to play in the context of thinking about domestic violence and abuse, and the expansion of how violence is conceptualised within domestic violence and abuse is long-standing. It now incorporates not only physical assault but also emotional, social, and financial abuse. Coercion and control come in many forms and that is now better reflected in official definitions, with use of the term domestic abuse better reflecting that expanded definition. In the context of studying migration and asylum, the place of violence requires a little more explanation; whilst its role within climate warming and other ecological crisis necessitates an even broader framing of what constitutes violence. The framing of violence that allows a linkage between those three sets of events, and that sees them as aspects of the broader appearance of violence within the maintenance of modernity, is one in which violence is seen not just as a singular explosive event or moment, but more as a continuous process of attrition. An unfolding of violence that might even be imperceptible in human terms in the case of violence against the environment: the millennia-spanning half-life of radioactive materials for example, or the decades long cycling of carbon and methane between atmosphere, land, and ocean. This altered perception of violence is articulated by Rob Nixon (2011):

> Violence is customarily conceived as an event or action that is immediate in time, explosive and spectacular in space, and as erupting into sensational visibility. We need, I believe, to engage a different kind of violence, a violence that is neither spectacular nor instantaneous, but rather incremental and accretive, its calamitous repercussions playing out across a range of temporal scales.
>
> (p. 2)

Nixon is mainly concerned with how the slow violence of environmental degradation and climate change is most frequently enacted upon countries and communities that have the least access to political and economic power within the neo-liberal global order. Through outsourcing, silencing, and intimidation, the effects of such slow violence become easy to turn away from and ignore. Especially for those protected by intersecting privileges. Slow violence is therefore a powerful expression of systemic violence. This becomes evident in thinking about the appearance of intergenerational trauma within the 21st century, as it appears in response to colonial violence and the use of slavery during the 18th, 19th, and 20th centuries. A similar process of slow violence continues to take place in the service of modern capitalism's need for cheap labour and the removal of environmental protections – mostly, but not exclusively confined to, the global south – and which will therefore continue to create trauma for many generations to come. In addition to the trauma that moves between and across generations, I would suggest that there is the appearance of a form of vicarious trauma that arrives as a consequence of witnessing slow violence at a distance, and that this acts as a partial explanation for the psychological pain and anxiety that is increasing as the climate crisis becomes more visible and manifest to more people (Doherty, 2015). Again, there is the need here to take account of how that visibility and manifestation differs between those parts of the world that have been living with environmental violence for many generations, and those parts just recently becoming consciously aware of it. Whilst most attention is given over to environmental violence, Nixon (2011) also considers slow violence as being manifest in other ways, entreating the reader 'to account for how the temporal dispersion of slow violence affects the way we perceive and respond to a variety of social afflictions – from domestic abuse to posttraumatic stress' (p. 3). Nixon takes an intersectional approach to thinking about the role of gender and race within environmental violence. The *Green Belt Movement* of Kenya, cofounded by Wangari Maathi, is given as an example of how racism, as expressed through resource exploitation and debt loading, coincides with the attempt to sideline women's experiences and voices by male-dominated political elites. Repeatedly, attention is drawn to the silencing of the dispossessed that is embedded within the actions of NGOs from the global north, and global financial organisations such as the World Bank, as they intervene within the global south in the name of both the conservation of nature and socio-economic development. When considering how environmentalism is frequently regional or national in focus, and concerned purely with the preservation of pristine non-human spaces, Nixon notes how '[a]ll too often, we are left with an environmental vision that remains inside a spiritualized and naturalized national frame' (p. 238). Amongst all of these critiques is a call for environmental thought, as it frequently appears within a white and western tradition, to learn from post-colonial writers about the intersections of injustices upon people and place that span generations and borders. It is this dispersed and systemic view of slow violence that makes it a useful lens through which to consider the violence that underpins the issues that this chapter and the next is concerned with.

Making environmental slow violence visible through acts of writing is where Nixon identifies one way to bring to light the expression of slow violence and its impact upon society. Likewise, Julietta Singh identifies those forms of literature that seek to critique global social and environmental injustices without succumbing to the urge to dominate and master those injustices (Singh, 2018). Both Nixon and Singh reference Indra Sinha's novel *Animal's People* (Sinha, 2007), which imagines a fictionalised account of the Bhopal disaster of 1984 and its impact on the lives of the Indian city afterwards, including the tragic failure to find justice and accountability within a globalised system that locates toxic and poisonous industries in places that are either least able to resist them, or least able to recover from their long-lasting toxic effects. *Animal's People* explores the category of 'human,' where that category is placed under stress by a lack of care and attention at an institutional and state level, but strengthened through familial and communal love and care. *Animal's People* is one example of fictional literature being used to bring forward and centre those formations of slow violence that are ignored and silenced. Similarly, Andreotti's analysis of the problems of modernity expressed through the image of the crumbling house sustained by violence, arrives at a position where a call to use imagination as a way of finding routes towards other futures appears. Andreotti states that 'if the architectures of existence that support the maintenance of the house are premised on continued violence, then we must re-imagine our existence if we want the violence to stop' (Andreotti et al., 2018, p. 29). From an art therapy perspective, in addition to the imaginary potential of the textual can be added other forms of creative expression, such as the making of visual images and objects.

In thinking more specifically about domestic abuse, linking the use of imagination and creativity with thoughts of the future resonates with philosopher Susan Brison's account of how she used her own subjectivity to make sense of her traumatic experience of rape and attempted murder (Brison, 2002). When trying to recover, Brison discovered that her training within the Anglo-American tradition of philosophy, with its focus upon positivism and rational analysis, did not assist her in the process of the 'remaking of the self after trauma' (p. 68). It was only when she began to consider personal narratives and autobiographical stories to be epistemologically valid that she was able to begin to make sense of her trauma and to start to construct for herself a different future. At one point in her account, she introduces the idea of postmemories and prememories of rape to suggest that the socialisation of young girls is heavily influenced by stories and images of abduction and rape, which in turn shapes feelings of fear and alters behaviour. Brison acknowledges this as being a controversial proposal, in terms of how it suggests limited agency in the face of strong cultural messages, but is one that she believes leads to a paradoxical situation in which causality becomes reversed. Brison expounds her position in the following way:

> Memory follows time's arrow into the past, whereas anticipation, in the form of fear or desire, points to the future. So how could one possibly remember the future? One way of trying to make sense of this paradox is to note that fear is a future-directed state and that it is primarily fear that is instilled by postmemory of rape. The backward-looking postmemory of rape thus, at every moment, turns into the forward-looking prememory of a feared future that someday will have been – a temporal correlate to the spatial paradox of the Mobius strip, in which what are apparently two surfaces fuse, at every point, into one.
>
> (p. 88)

The condition is one in which expectations of the future, informed as they are by the collective and personal recollections of past events, become fused together. The suggestion here is that traumatic experiences, both remembered and imagined, exaggerate this fusion of past and future. Brison is writing specifically about her experience of rape, but widens her argument to incorporate trauma generally. It is therefore legitimate to consider that a similar process forms part of the experience of other forms of violence, such as political violence and domestic violence.

Brison's response to her own sense of a damaged self is to make use of the telling of, and listening to, stories of trauma. She accepts that the recalling of stories of trauma risks wounding the listener, but sides with the view of Emmanuel Levinas (1996 cited in Brison, 2002) that there is an ethical need to recall and tell those stories. Brison proposes that it is through the acts of narrating stories that it becomes possible to live a future that is not limited by the past. The capacity of storytelling to contribute to differently imagined futures has qualities that appeal to a psychotherapeutic perspective of healing:

> It is only by remembering and narrating the past – telling our stories and listening to others – that we can participate in an ongoing, active construction of a narrative of liberation, not one that confines us to a limiting past, but one that forms a background from which a freely imagined – and desired – future can emerge.
>
> (p. 99)

The collective and creative qualities of telling and listening to stories emerges strongly here, and the reference made to desire resonates with how Stoetzler and Yuval-Davis (2002), whose work on situated imagination was introduced in Chapter 3, propose that there is the capacity for imagination to be turned towards ideas of pleasure and desire. The suggestion is made that any imagined emancipatory or egalitarian future needs to be inclusive of experiences of both pleasure and joy. This will become more evident as examples of imagination within the practice of a social action approach to art therapy, and within arts-based research, emerge in this and Chapter 5.

A collection of ideas also introduced during Chapter 3 that has relevance at this point of the discussion is Ann Murphy's (2012) examination of the appearance of imagination and violence within those philosophies and feminist actions that have an emancipatory objective. Murphy observes how the language of identity has been critiqued for its use of violent imagery, such as references to antagonism and division between the visible and the invisible, or the critique that '[s]ome see empathy as a necessary moment in the authentic recognition of others; but certain critics of phenomenology view empathy as a possessive gesture grounded in the conceit that one has access to another's experience' (p. 48). Rather than an argument being made that acts of making the hidden visible automatically provide access to previously concealed experience, which in turn enables empathy and emancipation, there is a questioning of how access to knowledge assumes that this then gives access to unmediated experience within a politics where visibility is synonymous with validation. From reviewing philosophies of identity, Murphy arrives at a position in which the division between visibility and invisibility is replaced with an acknowledgement of plurality and unintelligibility. This requires occupying a place of vulnerability and some renunciation of the link between knowledge and power. Unknowing and vulnerability do not fit easily with the sensibilities of modernity, predicated as it is upon mastery of the unknown and the hidden. A similar questioning of assumptions made about visibility appears in Thom Davies' response to Nixon's reference to the unseen within patterns of slow violence and the attempt to address that through writing (Davies et al., 2017; Davies, 2019). Agreeing with Nixon's general analysis of how environmental slow violence works, Davies states that '[i]n a pattern that is repeated the world over, environmental risks are commonly placed in the path of least resistance, near communities with the smallest reserves of political, economic, and social capital' (2019, p. 8). Nixon's conclusions are however reframed so that the 'out of sight' becomes 'unseen by some'; in the same way that it is more accurate to reframe the 'hard to reach' as the 'easy to ignore' (Escobar et al., 2017). The conception of visibility has as much to do with those doing the seeing as those seen; the level of visibility and invisibility depends on who is doing the seeing. The implication, from this and Murphy's observation, is that there is a need to question the assumptions about what can be achieved in any act of emancipation where there is reference to 'bringing to light' or 'making visible.' This raises the question of if and how the arts might aid visibility, and has profound implications for both art therapy and arts-based research. An assumption cannot be made that visibility is possible, or that it inevitably leads to empathy or emancipation. The reader or observer of such revelations has to question their responses to what they are presented with in a process of reflexivity.

Thoughts about violence and the remaking self make contact with ideas introduced in Chapter 3 about belonging and imagination, when attempting to understand, and respond to certain experiences through arts-based processes. These experiences are asylum and migration, and domestic violence and abuse. It is to these that I now turn, primarily through articulating my own involvement with arts-based processes of understanding and responding to these experiences as lived by other people.

Asylum and migration

Building upon qualitative research that investigated the role of bilingualism and translation within art therapy (Bird, 2011), I became involved with an Arts and Humanities Research Council funded network, *Making the Connections: Arts, Migration and Diaspora*. This network was co-ordinated by sociologist Maggie O'Neill and social geographer

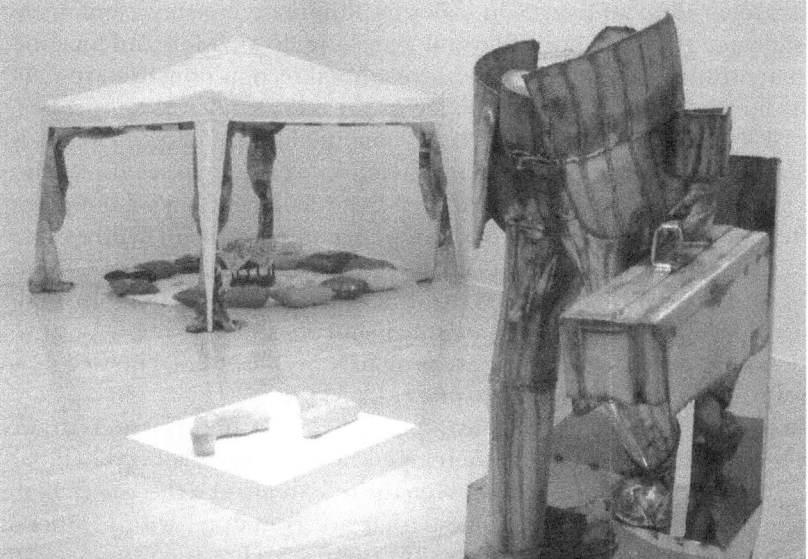

Figure 4.1 A sense of belonging, January 2009 (Photo by Jamie Bird)

Phil Hubbard, who were based at Loughborough University at the time, and used the arts to investigate experiences of migration and settlement within the midlands region of the United Kingdom. This network, through the production of a public exhibition titled *A Sense of Belonging* that took place at the *Bonnington Gallery*, Nottingham in January 2009 (see Figure 4.1)[1], as well as more traditional academic texts, sought to challenge common perceptions and stereotypes that existed within popular press and media about refugees and asylum seekers (O'Neill, 2009; O'Neill, 2010; O'Neill and Hubbard, 2010). The methodology employed within the *Making the Connections* network was one that made use of what O'Neill refers to as ethno-mimesis. Ethno-mimesis brings together ethnography, participatory arts, and participatory action research in order to create a space in which the arts can be used by participants to represent their life worlds in a way that captures the sensuousness and emotional quality of everyday life. This includes that which is celebratory and playful. It is a method that is primarily relational. O'Neill (2010) states that mimesis is used in this instance 'to express not the imitative dimension of social life but rather as sensuous knowing, the playful, imaginative and performative relationship we have to each other and to cultural forms and processes – indeed, to culture' (p. 99). It values participants' expertise as co-creators of knowledge and aims to engage the imagination of participants, researchers and audiences in order to illuminate injustices and make visible marginalised lives, whilst also seeking 'to envision and imagine a better future based on a dialectic of mutual recognition, care, respect for human rights, cultural citizenship and democratic processes' (p. 100). It is a method in which the imagined future of participants is considered to be as worthy of investigation as their past and present. It is a methodology I witnessed first-hand as having an empowering effect upon participants. It is also a powerful example of synthesising academic research with the principles of social justice, or what O'Neill refers to as performative praxis, within which the production of knowledge is viewed as having the explicit purpose of making a positive difference to participants' lives, primarily because that knowledge is produced *with* and *for* participants.

The way in which O'Neill uses participatory action research draws attention to those principles developed by Orlando Fals-Borda (1999) that attempt to close the gap between the researcher and the researched, such that assumptions and biases that are contained within official histories and narratives – and within the researcher themselves – are actively addressed and challenged. The researcher is open to being changed by their engagement with individual participants and communities. This is a reflexive position that asks researchers to think carefully about their own intersecting privileges and to how their own sense of belonging is constructed. This reflexive position is one that resonates with how social action and social justice has been thought about within previous chapters. In a contemporary sense, it supports attempts to decolonise practice and knowledge by observing how aspects of belonging and identity such as race, gender, sexuality, and mental and physical health are hidden or shown, and recognising that where how those aspects are constituted is taken for granted, they become ideological and hegemonic. Research, in this framing, is not an apolitical act, nor does the researcher sit within a vacuum, sealed off from that which is being researched.

Coming from an art therapy perspective, my own participation in the *Making the Connections* network involved the organisation of a day of seminars and workshops focussing on the therapeutic features of working with the arts, which formed part of a wider series of seminars and workshops hosted across the East Midlands, United Kingdom. By drawing attention to the therapeutic features of the arts, colleagues from the *Therapeutic Arts* subject area at the *University of Derby*, and myself, wanted to address both the benefits and the risks involved in asking people to explore complex, and often emotionally charged, topics through the use of non-verbal means of expression, where embodied responses and unconscious impressions are easily evoked. We addressed the need to consider how to emotionally support participants, researchers, and artists when working with a topic such as migration and refuge. The value of supervision was highlighted, and a critical view was presented of how the label 'posttraumatic stress' can make assumptions about how individuals respond to crisis, when it does not take account of cultural differences associated with what is valued as important to a person's sense of wellbeing and resilience.

In addition to the hosting of that event, my main involvement in the network was related to the accompanying participatory arts project *'Towards a Sense of Belonging'* and the subsequent exhibition held at the Bonnington Gallery, Nottingham. Reflecting upon the purpose and outcome of this arts project, O'Neill (2010) writes that:

> The arts practice communicates what belonging means to those participating in the research, exploring their experiences and feelings about home, dislocation, place making, belonging and friendship. The arts practice shows what it is like to live in Nottingham, Derby, Leicester and Loughborough for new arrivals as well as highlighting the perilous journeys people had made to seek freedom and safety from nations including Zimbabwe, the Democratic Republic of Congo, Iraq, Iran, Eritrea, Albania, Turkey and Afghanistan. The emotional and physical impact of those journey's, and the experiences of 'double consciousness' and being 'home away from home' are represented, alongside the rich cultural contributions and skills migrants bring to the region's cities, towns, cultures and communities.
>
> (p. 151)

An essential aspect of the purpose of the project was to represent the process of leaving one home, migrating across borders, arrival, and the establishment of a new home within a new community. What emerged was that those migrating into existing communities contribute to the way in which those same communities change over time. Communities are pluralistic and hybrid spaces, into which migrants introduce new practices, and from which migrants adopt and adapt existing practices. Communities can be both physical and virtual. Communities are dynamic, alive, and strengthened by the arrival of new migrants. They are also contested spaces within which those who belong are contrasted with those who do not, and where the very notions of belonging and of being bonded are formed and tested. If, as proposed in Chapter 3, belonging is intersectional, then the idea of community has to be one that is multiple and varied, and that can accommodate both pleasure and discomfort. As O'Neill identifies, the very concept of what constitutes a community is contested and prone to being used for political purposes; thus, within the context of when the project was being designed and implemented, the UK *New Labour* government was implementing an understanding of community that incorporated both a centralised approach to setting agendas and one that promoted participation at a local level. This was done in order to manage ideas of integration and national citizenship in the light of newly widened freedom of movement across the European Union (EU), and fears about national security following terrorist attacks in the early 2000s. Communities became places of governance and control.

In contrast to a centralised approach that dictates what citizenship entails, is a radically pluralistic approach, within which the emancipatory promise of equal citizens is balanced by an acknowledgement of variance that takes account of all aspects of the person. Thus, '[c]itizenship in a radical plural tradition involves an understanding of the individual as a socially situated self (not just a bearer of rights)' (O'Neill, 2010, p. 86). Reference to the situated self here is appealing because of it how resonates with the ways in which I earlier framed social justice, social action, and imagination. Taking into account a plural and situated understanding of citizenship and of community, *Towards a Sense of Belonging* showed that the experience of migration is a complex one, within which there are positive and negative components for both individuals and those communities that become the host of new migrants.

It is within the complex notion of communities that a participatory and ethno-mimetic approach to the making of art was employed by O'Neill and the *Towards a Sense of Belonging* project. Working together, artists, researchers, and those classed as refugees, asylum seekers, or migrants, used innovative methods to gather responses to notions of leaving, arrival, and belonging within the context of moving from one country to one another. The method involved walking together, talking, and taking photographs of places that resonated with those who have made those journeys between countries. The ethno-mimetic element of this process relates to how the emotional components of individual and collective experiences are made central to what the research is attempting to understand, with attention to how individuals and groups become emotionally attached to places, objects, other peoples, and groups. An arts-based approach to gathering data that pay attention to emotional attachments has much in common with art therapy.

The use of walking within a research context in this way draws upon the work of Sarah Pink (Pink, 2007b; Pink, 2009) and Misha Myers (Myers, 2010). Of relevance to how I have presented the unique qualities of arts-based research and imagination within earlier chapters, Pink brings to the use of walking in research aspects of sense-based ethnography that draw attention to all the senses in considering the emotional response and attachment to place. As well as what we see, what we smell, taste and hear is also important within responses to place, so that '*walking as place-making brings to the fore the idea that places are made through people's embodied and multisensorial participation in their environments*' (Pink, 2009, p. 77). This embodied response to place is

also a social process, within which walkers enter into a rhythmic dialogue with each other and the place they are traversing through. Pink
asks that researchers bring their whole selves to the process in a reflexive way. Myers echoes these themes, and in considering how examples
of walking as an arts practice, Myers observes that 'walks each involve
embodied, participatory and spontaneous modes of responsiveness
and communicability. Furthermore, they are conversive, activating and
inviting modes of participation that generate places and knowledge of
places through a conversational and convivial activity of wayfinding'
(Myers, 2010, p. 67). Such wayfinding might be preordained but it might
also be open to chance encounters, wrong turns, and becoming lost.
Incidentally, this multisensory and social aspect of walking, coupled with
the opportunity for the appearance of the fortuitous, resonates with
the way in which those therapists who base their practice out of doors
frequently describe their work (Atkins and Snyder, 2018; Heginworth
and Nash, 2019; Rust, 2020).

My own experience of taking part in walks as part of the *Towards a
Sense of Belonging* project, as well as demonstrating the embodied, multisensory and convivial aspects of the method highlighted how this way
of doing research fuses the past and present. There was a sense that
we were considering how this place we are in here now, reminds us of
another place back then. As an example, whilst walking with a young
man who had arrived from the Kurdish region of Northern Iraq, we
encountered the Derwent River as it flows through the city of Derby. We
stopped and took photographs. The river was a reminder for the person
I was walking with of their journey from Iraq to the United Kingdom. A
journey that often entailed the crossing of rivers. These were crossings
that not everyone survived. Whilst I did my best to be an attentive and
empathic witness of this memory, the horror of that experience can only
ever be partially imagined. Another example: we came across an area
in Derby made up of modern warehouses and car showrooms. The kind
of seemingly non-descript and anonymous places that many towns contain. This became a trigger for a memory of such spaces within the town
in Iraq that my walking partner had left behind. This was an encounter
that had a sense of longing, as well as a sense of discovering the familiar.

Other walkers took different routes in Derby and other cities.
Collectively, the photographs and the words used to describe them
acted as instigators for the next stage of the methodology, which was
to create maps. These maps were ones that layered together the physical and the emotional, the present, and the past. This meant that a
visual representation of the walk taken in the present made note of
those places that had resonance not only with those places left behind,
but also those places encountered on the journey between countries.
As the examples I have given above demonstrate, every physical place
has an attendant emotional tone. The maps therefore acted as ways of

bringing together on the page the mimetic and sensory qualities of the stories told of leaving, travelling, and arriving. From these maps, further group-based conversations evolved about the experience of migration and of seeking refuge.

Taken together, the photographs and memories that emerged from the walks, the maps, and the conversations, provided a rich source of knowledge for all those involved. This knowledge provided source material form which was constructed the artistic objects and performances that went on to form the *Towards a Sense of Belonging* exhibition. These objects and performances were co-created by migrants, researchers, and community artists. The group I was part of decided to create a representation of both the journey to the United Kingdom and the community activity that was formed after arrival. We created a miniaturised version of a shipping container of the sort used to move people across borders, though big enough for someone to crawl inside. Into this was placed objects that might be left behind in such a container: water bottles; food wrappers; discarded clothes; diapers and toys. We also created a soundscape of the kinds of noises that might be heard from within a shipping container: the noise of diesel engines; the bustle of a busy port; the laughter and tears of children. We aimed to create a multisensory experience that represented something of what it might be like to be confined within such a small space, not knowing where you were or when you would be able to leave. Wondering even, if you would survive the journey. In contrast to the deliberately uncomfortable interior was placed a set of brightly coloured patchwork curtains at the entrance and exit of the container. Those curtains, which draw upon traditional textile techniques, represented the way in which a new and vibrant sense of community was being formed, in spite of the travails of such a perilous journey towards asylum. Together, the interior and exterior of the container spoke to the way in which a range of emotions connected to the experience of migration and seeking refuge can co-exist. It also illustrated how difficult memories might be contained in literal and metaphorical ways, and which form foundations for something more hopeful.

Together, the objects and performances prepared for the final exhibition formed a powerful representation of the lived emotional experience of being a refugee, seeking asylum in the United Kingdom, and of the process of forming part of, and contributing to, a community. Testimony from participants and audience members demonstrated the power of an arts-based methodology, founded upon the principles of social justice and participation, to bring forth networks and knowledge that have the potential to change understanding and action. In her own analysis of the project, O'Neill (2010) writes that '[o]ur collaborations had real and tangible benefits for the participants (refugees, asylum seekers, artists, researchers, arts organizations) across the three strands of activity that included producing new knowledge, making connections, enabling "attunement," raising awareness and challenging myths and stereotypes' (p. 173). The benefit for me personally was gaining far greater appreciation of the emotional and practical complexity of refuge and asylum, and of how communities are evolving entities that mix the traditional with the novel as new groups and people settle and leave. I also gained an appreciation of how an arts-based and participatory methodology can create social change in a way that complements the psychological changes that art therapy can enable. Where they meet is in their appreciation of the emotional qualities of personal and collective experiences – an honouring of the mimetic qualities of experience.

Reflecting on the project ten years later, what I find disappointing and sad is that policies towards migration, refuge, and asylum in the United Kingdom seem to have deteriorated rather than improved. Public attitudes have stayed broadly the same, despite a significant decline in positive attitudes towards migration around the middle of the 2010s (Kaur-Ballagan et al., 2021), but existing UK government policies towards migration and the seeking of asylum have become more restrictive and draconian. That the explicit creation of a hostile environment towards migrants becomes a means of gaining political capital is a very real example of slow violence being enacted by the state. The reasons for this are complex and not unique to the United Kingdom, but beyond the scope of this chapter. What it is possible to say though is that this change in policy is one very real future response to the increase in migration that climate and ecological breakdown will entail over the coming decades and century. There are though other futures that can be entertained within the political imagination. Occupying and articulating those imagined alternative futures is one function of arts-based practices. The current state of political discourse around migration also says something about the importance of holding onto courage and hope, despite setbacks or the slow pace of change, and this is a fundamental position to occupy when it comes to responding to any crisis. It is especially important when contemplating climate and ecological crisis because of the all-encompassing scale of the crisis.

That need to maintain courage and hope in the face of uncertainty and disappointment is observed in accounts of art therapy being applied at an earlier point in the journey of migration. The *Artrefuge* project involves art therapists working within the refugee camps at Calais, France (Lloyd et al., 2018). It is framed as one point along a horizontal line that forms a path between countries and homes. Where the *Sense of Belonging* project was located more towards the point of arrival and settlement, *Artrefuge* is located at an earlier and more precarious point of the journey, where any emerging sense of safety or sanctuary can be rapidly blown away by actual winds, and political winds such as violent police actions. Being in such a place requires resilience, and to that end Bobby Lloyd, Naomi Press, and Miriam Usiskin write that '[f]inding shelter from the rapidly changing political climate, rules and weather, has needed a constant process of adaptation on the part of the refugees and those striving to support them' (Lloyd et al., 2018, p. 182). Resilience though comes at a price, with trauma, self-harm, and suicide being frequent occurrences in refugee camps. Art therapy can only offer so much in the face of this, but what it offers is one way of staying with what is so dreadful, at the same time as 'allowing a possibility of looking at the experience in different ways, of being enabled to live alongside difficult experiences while allowing them to be formed into something that can hold meaning' (p. 179). Art therapy in this context is closer to disaster and crisis-relief.

How *Artrefuge* works is to offer a space in which groups of participants can use different art materials and found objects to explore their experiences of being in the camp or to explore themes such as home and security. It draws upon the Portable Studio approach to art therapy (Kalmanowitz and Lloyd, 2011) within which a temporary, but safe, space is provided, often located outside of permanent structures and making use of found objects. Beginning as a response to political conflict in the former state of Yugoslavia in the 1990s, this approach has expanded to find ways of delivering art therapy that explicitly addresses social injustices in ways that are not constrained by the need for permanent structures and institutions. The temporary nature of the physical external structure is supported by internal structures: those of the art therapist and those of the person worked with, where the individual is considered 'as possessing internal resources rooted in experience, resilience and culture rather than being a powerless victim for whom the therapist alone holds the solutions' (Kalmanowitz and Lloyd, 2004, p. 108). From the examples provided of how the Portable Studio has been put into use, it is clear that those internal resources also exist powerfully at a group level. It is also clear that *Artrefuge* and the Portable Studio align with a social action and social justice approach to art therapy. Along with the *Sense of Belonging* project, they demonstrate how arts-based methods and interventions can work collaboratively with those seeking asylum within the context of therapy, research, and activism.

Domestic violence and abuse

Having witnessed first-hand how the arts can be used within therapies and research that have a social justice agenda, I was curious to know how this might work when transferred to the formation of a response to domestic violence and abuse. I had already been delivering some group-based art therapy for women who had experienced domestic violence and abuse, and the form in which this curiosity was explored was through the conducting of doctoral research between 2009 and 2015, supervised by Dr Becky Barnes (Bird, 2017). In that research, I set out to develop and evaluate a methodology that employed the arts as a means of documenting and representing women's experiences of domestic violence and abuse. Drawing upon an epistemology that values imagination and emotional experience, the methodology I employed involved small groups of women who had experienced domestic violence and abuse making visual images that represented their responses to thoughts and feelings about the past, the present, and the future within the context of their experiences of domestic violence and abuse. A mixture of collage and easy-to-use drawing and painting materials were offered to participants to aid in the construction of images. Collage enables people to engage with making visual images in a tactile and layered way. Arts-based researcher Lynn Butler-Kisber (2010) considers that 'collage evokes embodied responses, and uses the juxtaposition of fragments and the presence of ambiguity to engage the viewer in multiple avenues of interpretation' (p. 103). Collage also allows for the tactile qualities of materials to be used in a way that enables a multisensory approach to the representations of memory, imagination, thought, and feeling. The aim was for each woman to construct a visual response to their experience of living with and moving away from domestic violence and abuse. Discussions about those images took place during and after their making, and each woman had the opportunity to speak about the whole process at the end of their participation.

The resulting data were responded to and interpreted by myself in order to allow common themes to be identified, with those themes being related to contemporary understandings of domestic violence and abuse as they appear within literature. Where Gregory Stanczak (2007) claims that the meaning within visual images resides in the responses participants or researchers have to them, rather than within the inherent properties of the images, Pink (2009) suggests that a researcher might approach visual or sensory data through making use of their own imagination and embodied experiences in a way that enables a corporeal engagement with data. Likewise, Ephrat Huss (2013) argues that the analysis of visual images in research can be approached from a phenomenological perspective, in terms of acknowledging the unique interpretations that individual participants have about the images they have made. Huss also suggests that images can be approached from a social theory perspective, asking how the images might expose discourses of social knowledge and power. In this way, Huss argues that the 'analysis conceives of the art as a discourse that is both subjective and culturally embedded' (p. 23). In addition, Huss also proposes that where images are made within groups, then the interpretations made by the group form part of the analysis of images and reveal something of the social context within which the images were made. The approach taken by myself to responding to the images and words made by participants reflected the methodology set out by Huss. Following the collection of words and images made by women within the groups, time was devoted to immersing myself in what had been recorded. Firstly, by recording my responses to images in an unedited and reflexive way. Later, by grouping the stories as presented and told by participants together into themes using a process similar to that used within the phenomenological interpretation of the written or spoken word, whereby many individual points of interest are slowly grouped into larger patterns. Finally, those themes were related to existing literature about domestic violence and abuse.

The presentation of women's spoken and visual stories identified three major themes: the way in which the physical environment contributes to women's sense of freedom and harmony; the attempt to create a family and manage relationships and how support was sought and experienced during the pursuit of this idea; and the ways in which the women managed feelings around self-acceptance, self-belief and decision-making within their journeys away from domestic violence and towards the kinds of homes, relationships, and sense of wellbeing that they desired for themselves. These three themes I labelled in the following way: escape and harmony; relationships and social support; and agency and resistance. Together those themes reveal what I have to come to refer to as *transitional stories of domestic violence and abuse.*

Escape and harmony

Escape and harmony refers to how participants recounted their experiences of becoming aware of domestic violence, escaping and moving away from it, and their attempts to create a more harmonious life and home for themselves and their families – in the present and in the future. Some of this work was mental work, but mostly it was about the physicality of the participants' strategies to escape and achieve harmony. Those strategies and their articulation emerged in three ways. Firstly, the way in which women represented how they became aware of the effect of domestic violence upon their lives and started to move away from it; secondly, how the domestic environment, often in the shape of a new home, could be managed in a way that expressed a growing sense of control and agency; and thirdly, the natural environment becomes a literal and metaphorical form of escape and harmony. What was also observed was how strategies of survival and resistance that begin whilst living with domestic violence and abuse continue to inform imagined futures after leaving. Those strategies are embodied through everyday domestic acts and engagement with the built and natural environment.

An example of this appears in the three-dimensional image made by Jane (all names are pseudonyms). Figure 4.2 shows the way Jane perceived her ex-partners family controlling behaviour as being embodied

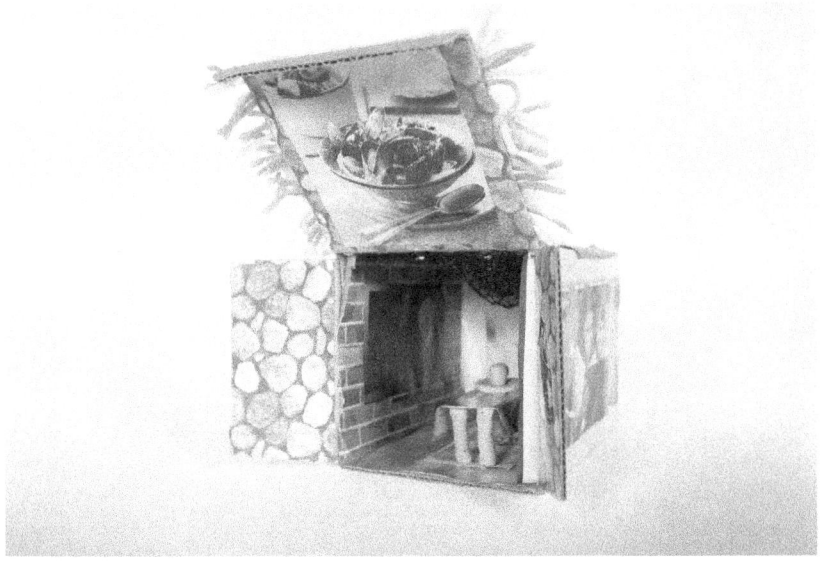

Figure 4.2 Jane's kitchen (Photo by Matt Howcroft/University of Derby)

in their style of kitchen that was primarily of brick and stone, and which she chose to reject when decorating her own kitchen. This even extended to the type of food cooked, where Jane rejected the style of cooking that had been imposed upon her by her ex-partner and his family. This is re-enforced where she states 'So it's me getting the confidence to just say goodbye to her and her standards and how she wants to live.' Another example is Figure 4.3, where another participant, Margaret, was comparing her sense of domestic comfort with the cold and stony nature of her marriage that had ended some years previously. Like Jane, Margaret was consciously managing her domestic environment as a form of self-determination and as a way of putting distance between herself and her past. The physical quality of materials (cold, warm, hard, soft, etc.) came to take on symbolic meaning for these women and other participants, so that we start to see how thoughts, feelings, and the physical properties of domestic spaces are interconnected.

As well as showing the management of the home in the present, there were examples of women thinking about how they would want their home to be in the future. Figure 4.4 shows an example of this where Anne represented her idea of a home she would want in the future. She described this image thus: 'the picture of me home is, is what I want for the future. I just want to be safe and secure and I've never had that in my, my life.' The important issue here is how, for Anne, the imagined future home is one that is not only safe and secure but one that can be something she has never had before. Elsewhere Anne spoke about her

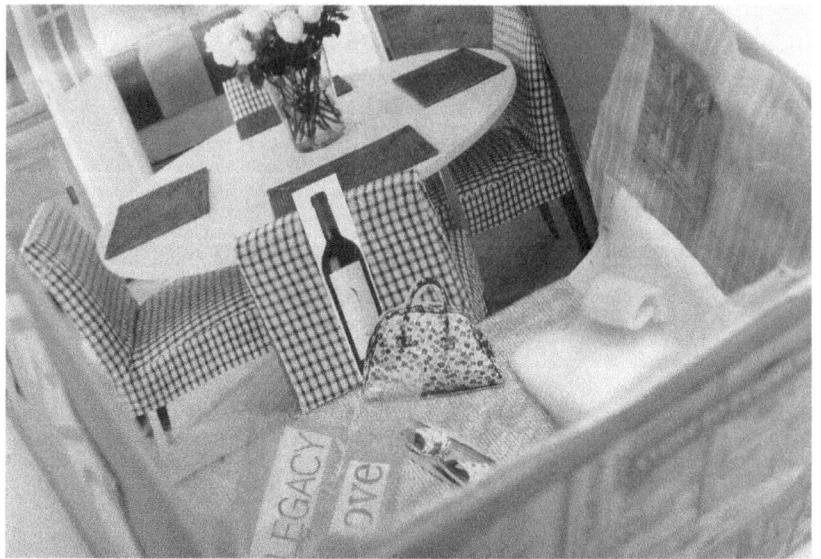

Figure 4.3 Margaret's domestic environment (Photo by Matt Howcroft/University of Derby)

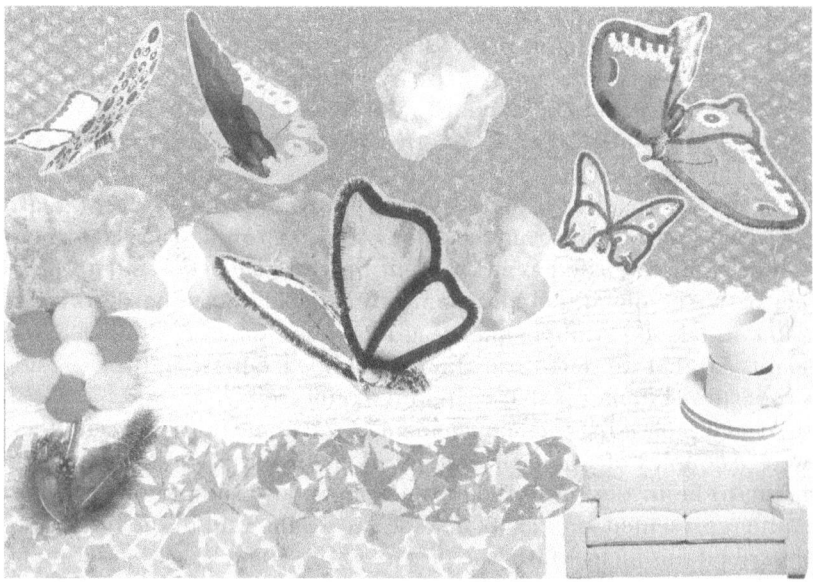

Figure 4.4 Carol's nature as freedom (Photo by Matt Howcroft/University of Derby)

childhood home being one of fear, but also spoke about her ideal home being similar in style to her childhood home. Relating these observations about the manipulation of the domestic space in the present and the imagined future home to literature, a number of pertinent connections appear. The importance of home and decoration to women who have experienced domestic violence has been identified by Hilary Abrahams (2010); in particular Abrahams writes that '[r]eplacing donated goods with items of their own choosing and redecorating their new homes enabled women to develop their sense of autonomy and build their confidence in making and taking decisions' (p. 44). The importance of the senses to everyday domestic life is explored by Pink (2009); for example, how the cleanliness of laundry is subjectively evaluated through sight and smell. In the images shown, the very simple and basic sensual qualities of decoration and of food contribute to the women's sense of autonomy: it is not just a new kitchen, it is a kitchen that feels warm and welcoming because its tactile qualities physically evoke those emotions, as well as having associations that run counter to the environment that is being rejected, and by association the relationship that is being rejected.

This intermingling of the sensual and the affective, the management of a physical environment, and the deliberate strategies of self-determination allows for the consideration of a key explanatory proposition that I wish to make in this book. It is an explanation that has its roots within the ideas introduced in Chapter 2 where I explored how imagination and embodiment were related to one another and pertinent to arts-based research and art therapy. In Chapter 2, I set forth the proposition that the link between thought and feeling, imagination, and reason was contained within the concept of embodiment, using various responses to the philosophy of Spinoza as a way of supporting that suggestion. Here, I want to introduce the work of neurologist Antonia Damasio (2000, 2004) and his development of the idea of the autobiographical self, as further support for that proposition. Damasio describes the autobiographical self in the following way:

> The autobiographical self is based on autobiographical memory which is constituted by implicit memories of multiple instances of individual experience of the past and of the anticipated future. The invariant aspects of an individual's biography form the basis for autobiographical memory. Autobiographical memory grows continuously with life experience but can be partly remodelled to reflect new experiences. Sets of memories which describe identity and person can be reactivated as a neural pattern and made explicit as images whenever needed.
>
> (Damasio, 2000, p. 174)

The important points to take away from this definition that are most relevant to my proposition are the plasticity of autobiographical memory, and the neurological basis for the mental images that make up autobiographical memory. An essential element of the way in which Damasio understands neurology is in the way that he places mental activity upon the foundations of the physicality of the brain and the body. Damasio believes that without a human body there is no human brain, and therefore no human mind and no human consciousness. Damasio (2004) writes that the current understanding of neurology allows for the suggestion '[t]hat the body (the body-proper) and the brain form an integrated organism and interact fully and mutually via chemical and neural pathways' (p. 194), explaining further that 'the images we experience are brain constructions prompted by an object, rather than mirror reflections of the object' (p. 201). Mental images are then, in this explanation, constructions: constructions that are framed by pre-existing responses the individual has had, including the affective, but also framed by socially accepted responses and emotions that the individual has been exposed to. Social responses such as shame, guilt, and sympathy are included here and this provides another way of considering the place of the body within a sociological understanding of experience.

A fascinating aspect of the theme of escape and harmony – in the context of thinking about climate and ecology – is how representations of nature appeared within all of the participants' images. There is a direct link between how the women employed representations of nature and how they employed representations of home: the physicality of the natural environment and the way in which nature contributed to feelings of freedom and self-determination mirrors similar associations with the home. The natural environment used as a metaphor for escape is evidenced within Figure 4.4. Whilst this image, made by Carol, was also about home, it is one in which nature is used very deliberately to act as a metaphor for feelings of peace, tranquillity, and freedom. There is in this image an intriguing joining together of the inside and the outside where the sofa sits amongst fields and sky. Of this image Carol said:

> And this one. Butterflies. Freedom. Clouds are breaking up, so giving me a clear sky. Done a flower because life is blossoming. Autumn leaves and you know. It was the time I was born really, autumn time and I just like it. It's so tranquil in a sense, and peaceful. But leaves being around and. . . you know, because their starting a new life, their breaking up the old and coming in with the new.

This image is also representative of how nature was used as a metaphor for transitions, and the image is a continuation of other images made by Carol that are positive and hopeful in tone and reflect her sense of finding a safe home and a safe partner.

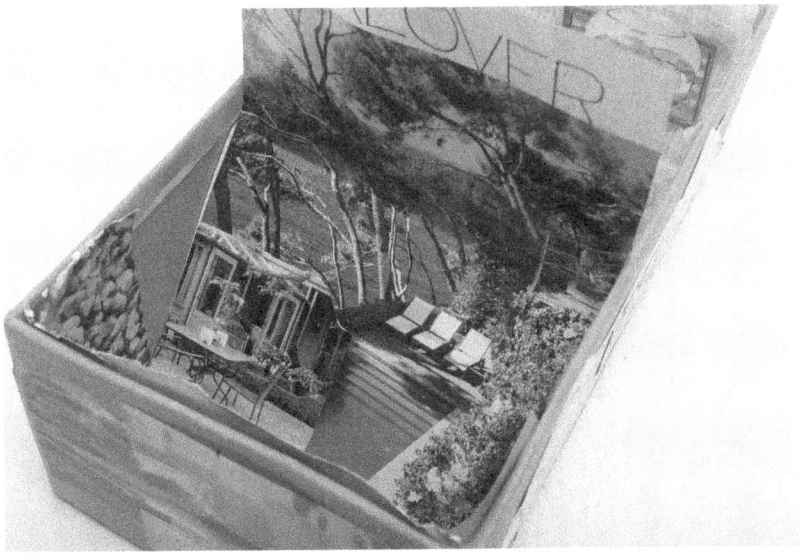

Figure 4.5 Carol's nature as freedom (Photo by Matt Howcroft/University of Derby)

The link between the use of nature within women's images, and the idea of escape and harmony, continued by way of reference to taking holidays or being immersed in nature Figure 4.5, was made by Margaret, and appears within the same three-dimensional box that contained her image of the domestic space (see Figure 4.3). Responding to this image, Margaret stated '*I like being surrounded by natural things … to sit and hear the sea … the tide and waves and lapping, it's just a wonderful sound.*'

The use of nature within images also allowed for the representation of complex feelings such as survival, resilience, and the ambivalence felt about choices made. This is best illustrated by images produced by Emma. Figure 4.6 shows a sun behind trees and the only comment Emma made about this image was that it represented her sense of 'not being able to see the wood for the trees.' It is an ambiguous image: Is the sun rising or setting? Is it an image of hope or of despair? It thus appears to continue a theme that Emma started earlier to do with feeling caught between darkness and light, and of feeling that she was in a relationship where, alluding to the lyrics of Bernie Taupin (John and Taupin, 1989), each partner was in their own separate world. Whatever the actual rational meaning of this image, it is an example of nature being used as metaphor for a feeling state; and of a wordless state at that.

Nature then was used by the women to represent different feelings; for some, it was a representation of relaxation or calmness; for some, it was used to denote self-determination or escape from control; for some, it was a metaphor for uncertainty. The representation of nature was also at times very literal, showing that nature was an environment

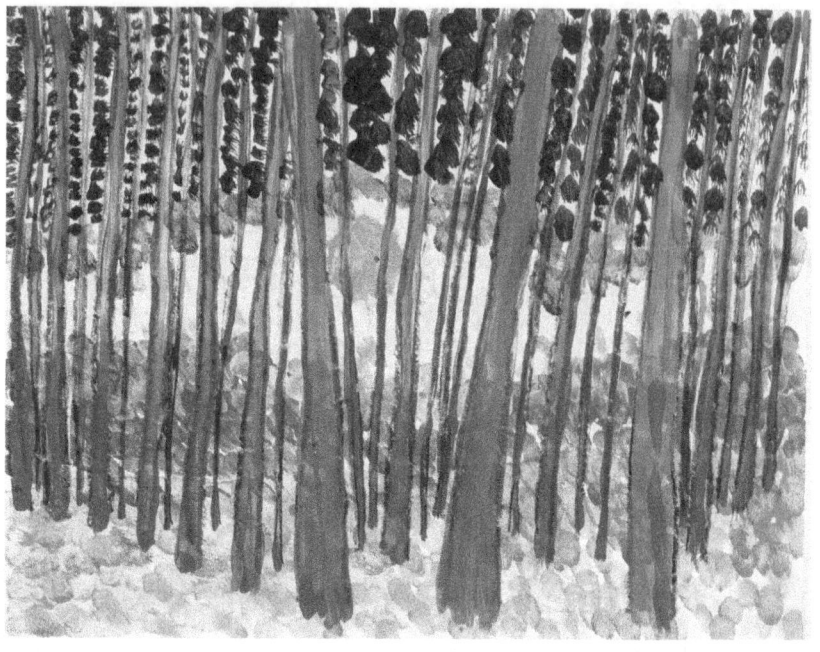

Figure 4.6 Emma's trees and sun (Photo by Matt Howcroft/University of Derby)

that some women desired to be in, including where it formed a component of being on holiday. In a similar way to how women had used representations of the domestic environment, representations of nature were a way of fusing together the literal, the metaphoric, the remembered, the imagined, and the desired. Similarly, the discussion had about sensuality and embodiment when thinking about the domestic environment, can continue when thinking about nature. My contention is that through evoking a sensual and embodied response, participants, in their employment of visual representation of real, imagined, and metaphoric spaces, did enable a sense of emplacement for themselves, and for me as a witness. The making of images and the employment of memory and imagination blurred the distinction between 'real' spaces and their visual representations; a distinction further blurred when participants were referring to those 'unreal' spaces that no longer existed or had yet to come into existence. This blurring or fusing of the real and the imagined is something that was observed both in women's representations of nature and of domestic spaces. Just as the sensual quality of women's representations of the domestic environment was considered with reference to Sarah Pink's (2009) investigation of perceptions of cleanliness, Pink's (2007b) exploration of walking interviews within visual and sense-based research has resonance here; as does similar research conducted by O'Neill and Hubbard (2010), in that whilst we never physically strayed from the rooms within which the research took place, in an imaginative sense the women travelled far and wide, to places they had been to and would like to go to.

Nature as a source of pleasure and comfort can also be related to the way in which the physical qualities of home were identified with achieving pleasure and comfort, and both appeared to contribute to the creation of a sense of harmony for participants. The search for harmony through nature can also, like the management of the home, be read as being part of a restoration narrative (Frank, 1995); whilst nature as a metaphor for uncertainty contributes to the representation of what Frank refers to as chaos narratives. As Frank (1995) states, '[t]o turn chaos into a verbal story is to have some reflective grasp of it' (p. 98). To this can be added that turning chaos into a physical image allows a similar transformation to occur.

A final point to be made about the appearance of nature in this context and that relates it to earlier discussions about imagination is to rethink what Genevieve Lloyd (1993) suggests about the place of nature and domesticity within western philosophy. In particularly its association within emotions, feelings, lack of rationality, and femininity. On the surface, it would seem that the way in which representations of nature were used by women within their images fitted with this contention, but if the engagement with nature is part of an active process that is both emotional and rational, then nature forms an important literal and symbolic space within the on-going management of the aftereffects of living with violence and control.

Relationships and social support

The theme of relationships and social support focuses upon the ways in which women explored the nature and quality of their relationships with others, especially with their immediate family, and of how those relationships aided and hindered their transition away from domestic violence and abuse. This emphasis follows on from escape and harmony, where it pays attention to the link between home and relationships, and in its use of the idea of escape and harmony as a way of understanding the women's representations of family. Family includes partners, children, and extended relations. This theme focuses then upon the relational and social aspects of women's stories. It also pays attention to how women encountered support offered by friends and family, as well as that offered by different agencies and services. The key finding here is that where services valued women's stories and involved them in decision-making they were viewed more favourably than when they made decisions for women, or failed to listen to their concerns.

As an example, it has been illustrated above in Figure 4.2 how Jane used the management of her home as a way of asserting control over her own life and as a way of rejecting the values of her ex-partner's family. Jane was working hard to create space and distance between how she conducted her life and how her ex-partner's family wanted her to behave. That work included management of the domestic space as well as her parenting choices. The box she created combines these two elements showing how the creation of home, for Jane, is intimately related to her parenting and her thoughts about being a mother. In the way that the box is constructed, that which is being moved away from is placed internally, whilst that which is being striven for is placed externally, so that here, the sense of what is internal is that which is to be hidden rather than being a place of retreat and safety. Elsewhere, Jane had said how she did try to keep her son in touch with elements of the culture of his father's family and with elements of her own culture. The box, with one culture being represented internally and one externally, is a visual representation of how she was managing that balance. What Jane's story also highlights is that domestic violence and abuse can extend beyond the immediacy of intimate partners to incorporate the extended family, who are able to assert control after the intimate relationship has ended and where children are involved.

Whilst Jane's story involved a sense of optimism in terms of having full access to her child and feeling like she was able to exert control over her role as parent, the more common experience represented by women during the research was that of estrangement from children, and the frustrations and hope of attempting to regain access to their children. Starting with Anne's story, we are presented with a particularly harrowing representation of what it means to be estranged from one's child. Like a number of other women, she responded to the idea of creating a three-dimensional image in the form of a box and used this to explore her thoughts and feelings about the relationship she had with her son. Figure 4.7 shows the inside of the box, and like Jane she chose to use the interior space of the box as a place within which to represent what was emotionally difficult to remember. An extract from a conversation between Anne and Jane during the final evaluation captures the essence of what Anne was trying to portray in the interior of the box: I were more pleased with the inside of the box than the outside because that really represents the past and the darkness, and, and, and . and . ya'know . to shut that away and think that's gone know.'

Within the interior of the box, she seemed to be trying to contain some of those feelings she had about her past and trying to come to terms with who she was, including her role as a mother. Crucially, this is the inclusion of a photograph of her son and the fact that she had placed this within the interior of the box, which for Anne represented the past. Anne spoke about having to leave her son behind in order to escape and the struggle ever since to regain access. On the exterior of the box Anne placed the words 'Come Home' and spoke about her hopes for a reunion but was unable to identify when or how this would

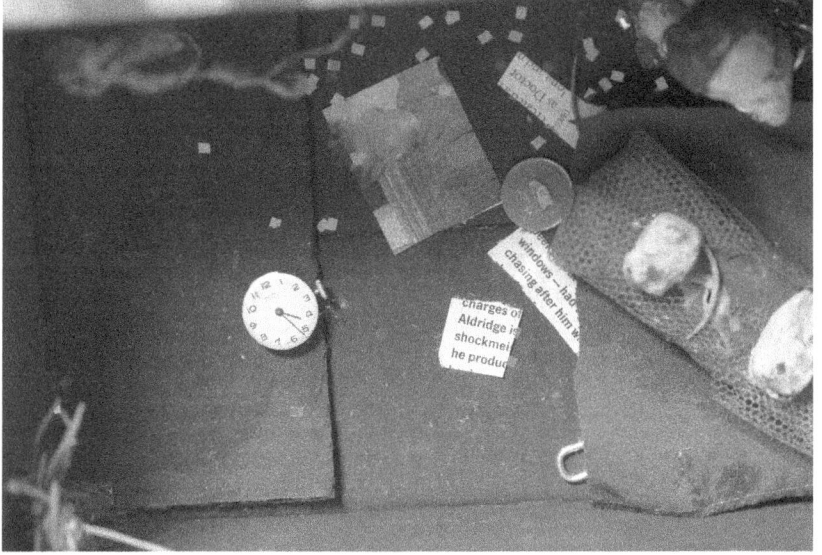

Figure 4.7 Anne's relationship with her son (Photo: Matt Howcroft/University of Derby)

happen. By using the words 'Come Home,' Anne introduces the theme of home being a potential space into which children might return. And for Anne, the material reality of what home was for her was as uncertain as the possibility of a reunion with her son. We have already seen how home can be as much an imaginary space as it can be an actual space; here that sense of home being an imaginary space is contributed to by the further addition of thoughts about children. For Anne, being a mother and part of family involved an element of return: a return of children, of the home, and of safety. I find that looking at the box Anne made, knowing how it refers to her feelings of loss for her son and the longing to find him, very difficult. It evokes a lot of sadness in me. This is to do with my own identity as a parent and my own experiences of not always having had the access that I desired. Such estrangement can feel very physical for me and I imagine that this is even more so for a mother. The box and the words 'Come Home' can be understood as a calling out in both hope and pain. In many ways this image, because of how it shows Anne's struggle to understand the estrangement from her son, comes close to being a chaos type narrative (Frank, 1995), whereby the telling and showing of a story becomes part of the process of trying to make sense of the experience that the story refers to.

In contrast to how Anne represented the relationship with her son is the way in which Carol represented the relationship with her children. Like Anne, Carol was not living with her children but could see a route to being able to do so. And like Anne, Carol viewed the idea of home as being a space that has the potential for the return of children.

Figure 4.8a shows the exterior of the box that Carol created. The words 'New Life' and 'Welcome Home' appear on the lid and the side of the box; neatly combining the sense of hope in the creation of something new with the desire for a return to something that has passed. Figure 4.8b shows a glimpse of the interior of the box, and it stands in marked contrast to what Anne created. Whereas Anne's was dark and fragmented,

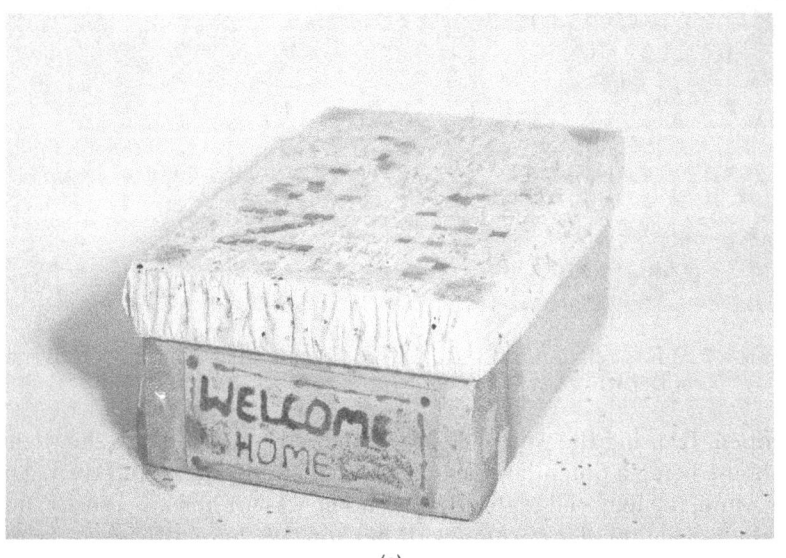

(a)

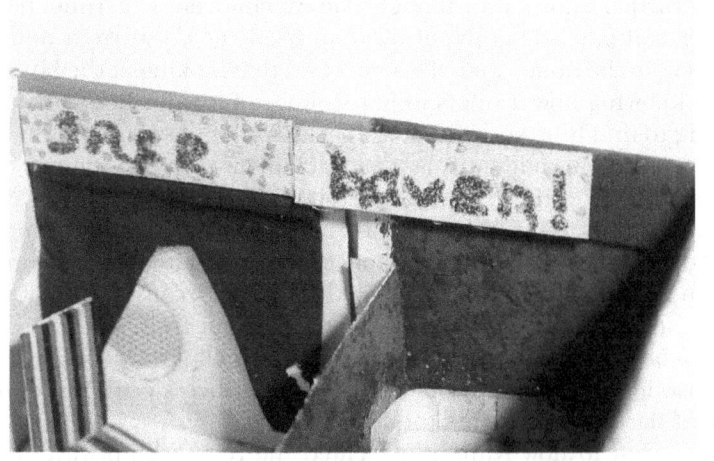

(b)

Figure 4.8 Carol's welcome home – (a) exterior and (b) interior (Photo by Matt Howcroft/University of Derby)

Carol's is brighter and more coherent. It represents how Carol had, in her new home, created a child's bedroom in readiness for the eventual and hoped for return of her children. This creation of a child's bedroom is a powerful symbol of hope and return, and of the home as a potential space within which a family can be re-formed or returned to. For Carol then, the making of the box was an important act that she was able to engage fully with, and its primary focus was upon how she was creating a 'safe haven' and a 'welcome home' for her children.

The importance of children within the stories told during the research confirms what Abrahams (2010) found in her interviews: that women placed children very centrally within their lives, basing many of their decisions upon the desire to parent their children in a way that was good for the children and countered the perceived negative effects that domestic violence had upon their children. As in the interviews Abrahams shared, there was also the appearance of guilt, anxiety, and determination, with respect to thought about parenting. The women with children who took part in the research were well aware of the need to provide a safe home for the children, now and in the future, and were prone to deep feelings of anxiety about how they would do this. Each of them had also experienced difficult relationships with Social Services in their journeys towards this, which undermined their confidence about being mothers, although not their determination to become part of a cohesive family. Hague et al. (2012), in an overview of the effects of domestic violence upon children, as well as noting the long-term psychological harm done to children witnessing domestic violence, critique the way in which mothers do not receive the support required to enable them to look after their children, or are hampered by bureaucracy, leading to a lack of trust between mothers and social workers. A key component of what a good supportive relationship was considered to be by the participants is the feeling of being seen and heard. The conclusion to be drawn is that where the women who took part in the research felt supported and understood they were better able to draw upon their own resources and make those changes that they deemed necessary.

In the stories that women where telling within this research, there was evidence to show that thoughts about the future family were contingent upon thoughts about the family of their own past and upon the social narrative of the good family. It was whilst exploring thoughts about children and family that I gained the sense that becoming a family and the return of a family were very closely related for some of the women. As shown by Anne and Carol, where they used the words 'Come Home' and 'Welcome Home' respectively, there was a very strong desire for a return to a former state. For Jane, there was less of a sense of return and a stronger emphasis upon becoming something new; which in her case was an independent and self-determining woman, who also happened to be a mother. For Jane, that sense of becoming was driven by her wish to create a home and style of parenting that was oppositional and resistant to what she felt had been imposed upon her by her ex-partner and his family.

Harmony, as has already been shown, is something that was in play for some of the women in the research, and the link between harmony and the physical home that emerged very strongly above can be applied to the ways in which the women with children thought about the relationships they had with their children. The uniqueness of what emerged within this research is how strongly related to each other the physicality of the home and the idea of family are for women who have experienced domestic violence and abuse. The home thus becomes a literal and metaphorical place within which there is the potential for the creation and recreation of an imagined set of supportive relationships.

Agency and resistance

Whilst the theme of escape and harmony was concerned with how the participants were managing their lives in the present and how they imagined their lives in the future, and the theme of relationships and support was focused upon the way in which those plans and desires were aided and frustrated through various types of relationships, the theme of agency and resistance pays closer attention to the internal thought processes and narratives that women employed when presenting stories about their transition away from domestic violence. This includes the way in which participants spoke about, and made images of, the process of making decisions; and the ways in which they managed their thoughts about how domestic violence had impacted upon their perceptions of self, their relationships, and their plans for the future.

A powerful metaphor that emerged within the research was that of a tightrope-walker, and how this represented walking a fine line between making right and wrong decisions. For one of the women, this meant decisions made about whether to leave her children behind or take them with her when she left her violent husband. For another, it was about decisions that she would have to make concerning her future employment and her desire for financial independence. This use of the metaphor of a tightrope-walker has parallels to the way in which the same metaphor has been used to describe how women who have been raped attempt to make sense of, and talk about, what has happened, in a way that honours their own unique experiences, whilst conforming to legally and medically accepted narratives about rape (McKenzie-Mohr and Lafrance, 2011). For McKenzie-Mohr and Lafrance, precariousness and doubt emerge in the telling of stories of sexual violence. For the women in this research, those doubts emerge in how they make decisions in response to domestic violence and abuse. What the tight-rope metaphor allows for is an appreciation of how the experience of doubt and uncertainty might physically and psychologically feel like. It is a powerful embodiment of a complex set of emotions that can leave women feeling in a precarious and vulnerable position. As indicated above, where those decisions will have an impact upon a mother's relationship with her children, these feelings are heightened further. The stories and incidents that women told and had played back to them centred on the balance between doubt and hope: doubts about decisions made in the past; doubts about decisions made now and the anxiety of having to make decisions in the future; and the desire to not have to make decisions because of the anxiety that it provokes. It was stated quite clearly that by its very nature an abusive relationship took away the women's trust in their own abilities to make decisions, even where hope for a better future was in existence.

The appearance of feelings about the decision-making process come together in one key image that was produced by Emma during the end of her participation Figure 4.9. This image was the culmination of many weeks of preparatory work; with Emma developing her ideas both in the group and away from it. Her on-going training in artistic skills aided her in the making of the image, and, as a consequence, it has an aesthetic sophistication that gives it extra significance in terms of viewer engagement. In her conversations about this image, Emma spoke about how it represented the choices that she was faced with and the anxiety that accompanied that need to make a decision. It was also an image that explored her acceptance of what had happened to her in the past, acknowledging the anger she faced and her ability to survive a violent partner. Running up through the centre of the image is the representation of a cross-roads sign that asks the question 'Which way?' On the left-hand side of the image is the appearance of those things Emma associated with her ex-partner that she had explored in other images earlier in her participation: shouting, swearing, anger, coldness, and cruelty. On the right-hand side are representations and words that show Emma's sense of survival and of how she had been affected by living with domestic violence, so that we see and read something about being battered, bruised, and 'Driving off the edge,' as well as being shown a representation of how Emma again drew inspiration from the lyrics of *I'm Still Standing* (John and Taupin, 1983). Dancing, music, art, sunshine, and a 'lucky white feather' contribute to that aspect of the image. Read in an anti-clockwise direction from the top-left of the image around to the top-right, the image can be seen to represent the journey that Emma had taken as she moved away from a violent partner. In one area of the image, towards the lower and central area is found representations of how Emma came to realise that she could not live with violence any longer.

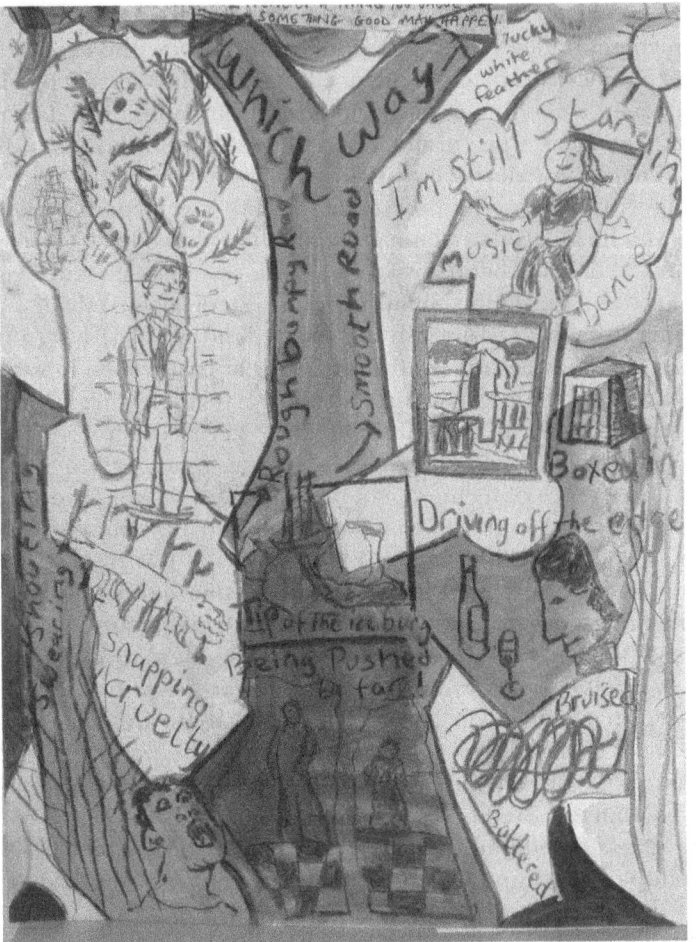

Figure 4.9 Emma's cross roads (Photo by Jamie Bird)

Agency is an important concept to explore at this point. Within domestic violence and abuse literature, it has a particular meaning. It is a key component of Liz Kelly's (1988) differentiation between the labels of victim and survivor. It is introduced by as a way in which women form 'distinctive internal definitions of self and situation and to develop problem solving and coping strategies to resolve the conflicts and to end the violence' (Lempert, 1996, p. 286). Agency can be both active and passive and can be considered to be in evidence where 'women [use] conscious decision making to take action, not only active behaviours (e.g., calling the police) but other actions that would be defined as passive (e.g., subordinating the self) in most theoretical schemas' (Campbell et al., 1998, p. 758). It is thus a term that gives value to any action a woman might take in response to domestic violence that is conscious and aims to keep them safe. With its inclusion of passivity as a conscious management strategy, it challenges social definitions of the passive victim of domestic violence. Whilst there was little in the way of women recounting how they moderated their partner's behaviour – with much of the agency that emerged within women's narratives referring to actions taken after leaving – an action like Emma's use of song lyrics shows how simple acts were used to gain a sense of self-expression when living with domestic violence and abuse, and after leaving.

What Figure 4.9 shows is how Emma had to work hard on maintaining her sense of having made the right decision in choosing to leave when she did. Emma was exploring the delicate balance between going forward with a sense of optimism and returning to a former state of fear. But that choice is not so much about choosing between staying away from a violent partner and returning to them, but more to do with uncertain feelings about the future: will it be a 'Rough and bumpy road' or a 'Smooth road'? Emma's image is a very complete image where it shows different aspects of a lengthy and on-going journey, incorporating thoughts and feelings about the past, the present, and the future. Whilst there is uncertainty, there are also signs of optimism, represented by signs of pleasure and joy. These include representations of music, dance, and art. The image is thus one that encapsulates a complete, although unfinished, journey away from domestic violence and abuse. Its attention to the uncertainty that surrounds making decisions is one that corroborates what has been observed within the narratives of women who have been controlled to such an extent that the making of any decision, after leaving a controlling and violent partner, is accompanied by both fear and anxiety (Abrahams, 2010). It also fits with the framing of domestic violence and abuse as being about power, coercion, and control. Figure 4.9, like the metaphor of the tightrope-walker, exhibits the kind of ambivalence that has been identified elsewhere (Campbell et al., 1998) as appearing within women's thoughts about what might happen in the future when contemplating and planning to leave a violent and abusive relationship.

What Emma's image, and other images made by other women, indicates is how the process of managing thoughts about the past are active, dynamic, and layered, and that they can be extended forward in time. It shows how there can be a conscious choice made as to how the past is allowed to shape the present and influence the future, so that the negative elements of the past can be actively resisted and a different, more hopeful future, actively imagined. What the proceeding themes have shown is how resistance and imagination are aided by the self-determining acts associated with the management of physical space and relationships. What Figure 4.9 suggests is that the transition away from domestic violence, and the attendant anxiety and doubt it generates, is also managed through the management of thoughts and images of the past, the present, and the future.

A statement made by Jane encapsulates very well the coming together of these ideas about the management of both internal and external factors and the management of the self through time. In talking generally about how she was working on creating a different kind of home and set of relationships, Jane stated that 'I couldn't move forward if I didn't look back.' The power and significance of Jane's words is that spatial ('move forward') and visual ('look back') metaphors come together in thoughts about the management of the self through time. On the one hand, reference is being made to the physical elements of moving forward in time, which can be taken as being representative of how the future was aligned so strongly to the physicality of home and place within many of the stories women constructed about their imagined futures. On the other hand, the reference to looking backwards hints at the psychologically internal process of reviewing the past; a process that Jane suggests is essential to the making of a life in the future. In a somewhat similar way, Carol spoke at one point about being in a better place that allowed her to look backwards more clearly. The 'better place' she referred to was not only physical but also emotional, and the ability to see the past more clearly was identified by Carol as a necessity if she was to regain access to her children. Taken together, Jane's and Carol's words about looking at the past in order to move forward provide spoken evidence that complements Emma's image (see Figure 4.9) about the interconnection between points in time within women's autobiographical stories and about their transition away from domestic violence.

Agency and resistance have been referred to here to help frame the internal mechanism women employed to manage the thoughts about the transition away from domestic violence and abuse. Agency has been introduced as conscious action that is both active and passive and that keeps women safe, with the suggestion made that agency is as much a feature of life after domestic violence and abuse as it is when living with domestic violence and abuse. Resistance shares something of the qualities of agency in terms of how it can be considered as part of women's management of domestic violence. It does though differ in one crucial component and that is in the way that it can be conceptualised as a collective, as well as an individual, response to domination. This claim is made in light of a view of domination being 'ossified relations of power' (Mclaren, 2004, p. 220), and an understanding of power being non-subjective and 'relational, existing only between and among persons, institutions, discourses, practices and objects' (p. 220). This view of power and domination, from a feminist perspective, can be applied to an understanding of patriarchy and gender-based violence; likewise, such an understanding means that it is only through collective resistance that freedom and liberation is possible. This is an understanding of resistance that challenges the view of domestic violence and abuse, its consequences upon women's health and wellbeing, and associated responses, as being only of concern to individuals and couples. Instead, it places that concern within the realm of the collective and the social. Such a view can be used to critique the language used to describe responses to domestic violence and abuse: whilst 'victim' and 'survivor' imply an individual response and level of accountability, resistance implies a collective and shared answer to domestic violence and abuse. This consideration of agency and resistance operating at a collective level will return in Chapter 5 when considering responses to climate crisis. Firstly, the topics and themes explored in thinking about asylum and refuge, and domestic violence and abuse, are brought together within the concept of transitional stories.

Transitional stories: part 1

Whilst the concept of a transitional story does have relevance in thinking about migration, refuge, and climate change, its genesis in my thinking, as shown above, comes from what I observed in those stories told by women who have experienced domestic violence and abuse (Bird, 2017, Bird, 2019). A transitional story, as it appears within domestic violence and abuse, is one that entails the representation of physical and emotional movement between places, movement through time, and changes in relationships. Together these transitions contribute to the ways in which women who have experienced domestic abuse perceive themselves and engage in tactics of agency and resistance. There are elements of transitional stories that contain acts of agency and control, and elements that highlight barriers to the achievement of goals and desired outcomes. A transitional story is one that encompasses the past, the present, and the future. It is a story that acts as a bridge between points in time and allows imaginative movement between those points. Transitional stories are extendable into the future and are heavily imbued with a sense of place and located within a social and political context; a context that is shaped by the social constructs of gender, race, class, and health. Within transitional stories, how women survived and escaped violence and abuse can be reframed as being about how they resisted that abuse and violence, with that resistance persisting into the present and on into the future. Resistance is manifested in states of mind, such as a determination to have a better life or to regain a sense of harmony. It is also manifested in a myriad of physical acts such as choices about internal decor, garden maintenance, choice of food, walks in the countryside, and other acts that help to form 'zones of safety' (Frohmann, 2005). Transitional stories show how those internal and external features worked together. It is this inter-twining of the mental and the physical, and the joining together of the past, the present, and the future that gives transitional stories of domestic violence and abuse their unique quality. Such stories contain aspects of the kind of processes that Susan Brison (2002) recognises in attempts to remake the self, following experiences of violence. They also contain what Vanessa May (2013) identifies as being important components of the relational self and social belonging: change; motion; and the importance of everyday social actions.

A transitional story, in its expression of multiple and layered points in time, allows for the simultaneous showing of different physical spaces, and the merging of memory and imagination. It gives tangible expression to the experience of living with and beyond domestic violence and abuse as something that is complex, uncertain, fragile, and ambiguous. It also makes manifest how agency is employed across time and is associated with both tangible everyday domestic acts, the intangible management of relationships, and the desire for escape and harmony. The fluidity of transitional stories, however, means that they can only ever offer situated and approximated truths.

The way in which the women in the research cited above most often expressed their acts of agency was through the management of relationships and engagement with the physical environment. An important finding of that research is that the various processes associated with the movement away from domestic violence are bound up with the physical environment, and that the embedding of the personal and the interpersonal within the physical environment stretches forward in time in a way that allows agency to be asserted and ownership taken of both the present and the future. The appearance of the physical and the temporal within transitional stories can be framed as stories that are situated in place (emplacement), within the body (embodiment), and in time (emplotment).

The concept of embodiment had already been identified as a strong guiding principle within the epistemological and methodological foundations of the research. What emerged from the women's stories was that not only was embodiment an appropriate concept to integrate into the research, but also how strong the sense of place was for many of the women; for this reason, an incorporation of the concept of emplacement became necessary. As Sarah Pink identifies, whereas embodiment relates to the interconnections between the mind and the body, emplacement refers to the multisensory integration of the mind, the body, and the environment. Pink (2009) argues that emplacement within ethnography means paying attention 'to the question of experience by accounting for the relationships between bodies, minds and the materiality and sensoriality of the environment' (p. 25).

A pertinent way in which to think about embodiment, within the contexts explored here, is in how Arthur Frank (1995, 2010) thinks through the role of the body within stories told about illness. What Frank refers to as the communicative body appears within the way in which quest narratives explore the narrator's communication of their confrontation with the contingency of the physical body. It appears also in the consideration of the way in which narratives speak of and for the other through testimonies of the suffering and recovering body, with Frank (1995) stating that '[i]llness stories are told by bodies that are themselves the living testimony; the proof of this testimony is that the witnesses are what they testify' (p. 140). Domestic violence and abuse very much include the physical body, either because of direct physical violence, the threat of it, or disruption to the relationship between victims of violence and their physical environments. Brison (2002) similarly highlights the connection between the body and the mind, particularly the disruption of that link following violent trauma; and whilst not as explicit as Frank in her incorporation of the body into explorations of survival and recovery narratives, Brison does speak about the process of *'physically remastering the trauma'* (p. 76). For Brison, this was achieved through self-defence training. Within the women's transitional stories, physical remastering was most obvious within their management of the material aspects of the home. It was also apparent within their engagement with the natural environment; an engagement that whilst being mostly of symbolic and metaphorical value, also hinted at how it offered an actual place to be physically present and away from the emotional pain of having lived with domestic violence. If, as Brison (2002) argues, violence disrupts the concept of the body, and that violence also exposes a sense of vulnerability that can be responded to with imagination, agency, and resistance, it is possible to think about transitional stories as exhibiting the corporeal vulnerability that Ann Murphy (2012) proposes as forming part of an emerging feminist ontology. Such a feminist ontology seeks to not only understand the vulnerability associated with violence, but also the vulnerability that comes about through acts of telling and showing. It is associated with the potential for care and compassion between individuals. Vulnerability following violence isolates the individual, whilst the sharing of that vulnerability counters that isolation.

Whilst the physical body did not figure strongly within the women's stories, the representation of the interaction and management of the physical environment revealed not only the embodied nature of their experience but also the emplaced nature of the women's stories. Emplacement is concerned with both corporeal and temporal movements, and corporeal movement was a strong feature within the women's stories where those stories represented a movement between homes or the desire to travel. Accompanying that representation of physical movement, movement through time featured strongly within the stories told. This temporal movement was implicit, in the sense that any story will imply a shift between points within a narrative; it was also explicit in those representations where women represented their thoughts about how they thought about the past, the present, and the future. For example, where women used images of clocks and watches this seemed to indicate feelings of ambiguity about the flow of events. This expression of time can be read as exposing an underlying metaphor of time being uncertain.

The women though, in their telling of narratives and construction of stories, were making attempts to extract meaning and impose an order upon their experiences of time. In this way, the agency that was expressed about their management of home and relationships can be seen as being repeated within the way they took control of the stories they told, and can be thought of as one expression of emplotment. Frank (2010) writes that emplotment means to take the 'brute sequence' (p. 137) of events and to find connections and purpose between different experiences and different points in time: '[t]o emplot is to propose a plot that transforms what are still incoherent things-that-are-happening into experience that has meaning' (p. 136). Emplotment is a relevant term to be using about the women's stories because it takes those feelings of disconnected and confused experience – including the very flow of time – and makes a coherent structure of them. Frank also identifies institutional emplotment as the imposition of institutional or group meaning upon individual experience. This form of emplotment seems strongly related to his earlier identification of a typology of narrative types that individuals either adopt or resist in response to illness. Within the women's stories, institutional emplotment made an appearance within the expression of their encounters with different services and within the appearance of wider social narratives about gender, home, and family. In the women's stories, there was both acceptance and rejection of institutional emplotment. For example, there was a strong association with the role of homemaker, whilst the role of passive victim or failed mother was strongly resisted. Either way, there was an active response to such forms of emplotment that was personal and political, emotional, and physical.

The sense of place and time being a structural, as well as a personal encounter that the foregoing discussions about emplacement and emplotment involve, can be related to Gillan Rose's (1993) thoughts about feminism and geography. Whilst Rose does not use the terms emplacement or emplotment, her exploration of the gendered body as it is represented within geography suggests that the terms fit with her understanding of how physical spaces are negotiated in gendered ways. This is expressed when considering the notion of time-geography:

Time-geography was adopted by some of the earliest feminist geographers, and it is not hard to see why: it recovers the everyday and the ordinary, and many feminists have argued that the mundane world of the routine is the real of women's social life in masculinist society. Examining the lives of women requires attention to the ordinary, to the unexceptional, because women are excluded from arenas of power and prestige.

(p. 22)

Time-geography draws attention to everyday tasks and activities and makes them a site for the expression of power and agency. It aligns with Pink's (2004, 2007a) attention to gender and domestic space within sense-based ethnography, and gives extra value to how the women in this study expressed their relationship with the home and domestic activities and to how Hilary Abrahams (2007, 2010) identifies women's desire to create new homes for themselves following experiences of domestic violence and abuse. The time-geography that Rose refers to is relevant because so much of how the women in the research highlighted here exhibited resistance, agency and recovery, emerged through the everyday acts associated with home and relationships with family and friends. It was also exhibited in their desire for those things in the future. Within this research, the concepts of time-geography, embodiment, emplacement, and emplotment all appear within the imagined futures that form part of women's transitional stories. What is observed is how transitional stories that are begun during the time of living with domestic violence continue through, and then beyond, the period of leaving and rebuilding. The transitional stories that women presented were inclusive of the body and of place, and allowed a representation of how agency, identity, and belonging changes dynamically through time. The imaginative, sensorial, and temporal qualities of the stories, with their inclusion of the future and their contingency upon interpersonal and structural forces, illustrate how transitional stories are both situated and embodied.

The value of seeking to understand the embodied and emplaced nature of experience within the study of domestic violence and abuse finds support where Maggie O'Neill (2008) writes that '[t]he texts, objects and images emerging from this work have the potential to enable us to experience, imagine the overlapping spaces and places of exile, both physical, mental and social – the embodied experience of exile, displacement and emplacement/belonging' (no page). O'Neill is here referencing the experience of exile, arrival, and settlement within stories of migration, and of how art enables an imaginative dialogue with both the emplaced and embodied nature of that journey. As already explored, belonging is a coalescence of the physical, emotional, relational, and political. Emplacement and belonging, observed within the experience of refuge and migration, can be transposed on to the experience of transitioning away from domestic violence and abuse. The sense of belonging identified within diaspora communities finds equivalence in the way women who have experienced domestic violence and abuse seek security and safety within the home, and within renewed and reclaimed relationships with family, friends, and those agencies that offer them support. Whilst there are similarities between the experience of refugees, asylum seekers, and those who have experienced domestic violence and abuse – the experience of being exposed to or witnessing violence; the sense of exile; the seeking of sanctuary; the oftentimes precarious and chaotic nature of daily existence; the hope and anguish of a return to what once existed; and the desire for a safe and harmonious future – the crucial difference is that those diaspora communities that are formed by refugees, asylum seekers, and economic migrants, will be larger and more tightly woven together than any community that emerges from the coming together of people who have experienced domestic violence and abuse. This is because domestic violence and abuse by its very nature isolates individuals and families, and keeps them hidden from view.

Summary

The focus in this chapter has been upon articulating how arts-based research, that includes an explicitly participatory and emancipatory component, has been helpful in better understanding experiences of refuge and migration, and domestic violence and abuse. Both have been identified as forms of crisis that disrupt belonging, self, and safety. Both entail processes and stories of transition. Understanding these experiences better is of value to researchers, those providing help and support to people in crisis, and most importantly – in the context of an objective of emancipation – those people who have lived through and with those experiences. It is that last element that provides a bridge to thinking about how arts-based research blends into art therapy, where there is the appearance of the possibility of participation being a transformative and therapeutic process.

Those aspects of belonging and of transitional stories that have been identified within accounts of domestic violence and abuse, and in accounts of seeking refuge and asylum, have much to offer how experiences of climate and ecological crisis are received and responded to. In Chapter 5, there is a detailed exploration of how a social action approach to art therapy can be usefully applied to responding to that crisis, with both sensitivity to belonging and transitional stories playing a part in that response. Transitional stories become adaptation stories where the place-based component of belonging is disrupted either in the present or in the near future.

Note

1 Further photographs of exhibition, by Aria Ahmed, available at: http://www.guardian.co.uk/society/gallery/2009/jan/13/sense-of-belonging-exhibition?picture=341562670 [accessed: 12/1/2022]

References

Abrahams, H. 2007. *Supporting Women after Domestic Violence: Loss, Trauma and Recovery*. London: Jessica Kingsley Publishers.

Abrahams, H. 2010. *Rebuilding Lives after Domestic Violence: Understanding Long-Term Outcomes*. London: Jessica Kingsley Publisher.

Albrecht, G. 2005. Solastalgia: a new concept in human health and identity. *Philosophy Activism Nature*, 3, 41–44.

Andreotti, V. O., Stein, S., Ahenakew, C. & Hunt, D. 2015. Mapping interpretations of decolonization in the context of higher education. *Decolonization: Indigeneity, Education & Society* 4, 21–40.

Andreotti, V. O., Stein, S., Sutherland, A., Pashby, K., Susa, R. & Amsler, S. 2018. Mobilising different conversations about global justice in education: toward alternative futures in uncertain times. *Policy and Practice: A Development Education Review*, 26, 9–41.

Atkins, S. S. & Snyder, M. A. 2018. *Nature-Based Expressive Arts Therapy: Integrating the Expressive Arts and Ecotherapy*. London & Philadelphia: Jessica Kingsley Publishers.

Bird, J. 2011. Towards Babel: Language and Translation in Art Therapy. *In:* Burt, H. (ed.) *Art Therapy and Postmodernism: Creative Healing Through a Prism*. London: Jessica Kingsley Publishers.

Bird, J. 2017. Art therapy, arts-based research and transitional stories of domestic violence and abuse. *International Journal of Art Therapy*, 23, 14–24.

Bird, J. 2019. "The Eye of the Beholder": Encountering women's Experience of Domestic Violence and Abuse as a Male Researcher and Art Therapist. *In:* Hogan, S. (ed.) *Arts Therapies and Gender Issues: International Perspectives on Research*. London: Routledge.

Brison, S. J. 2002. *Aftermath: Violence and the Remaking of a Self*. New Jersey: Princeton University Press.

Butler-Kisber, L. 2010. *Qualitative Inquiry: Thematic, Narrative & Arts-Informed Perspectives*. London: Sage.

Campbell, J., Rose, L., Kub, J. & Nedd, D. 1998. The voices of strength and resistance: a contextual and longitudinal analysis of women's responses to battering. *Journal of Interpersonal Violence*, 13, 743–762.

Damasio, A. 2000. *The Feeling of What Happens: Body, Emotion and the Making of Consciousness*. London: Vintage.

Damasio, A. 2004. *Looking for Spinoza: Joy, Sorrow and the Feeling Brain*. London: Vintage.

Davies, T. 2019. Slow violence and toxic geographies: 'Out of sight' to whom? *Environment and Planning C: Politics and Space*, 40, 409–427. Available: https://doi.org/10.1177/2399654419841063.

Davies, T., Isakjee, A. & Dhesi, S. 2017. Violent inaction: the necropolitical experience of refugees in Europe. *Antipode*, 49, 1263–1284.

Doherty, T. J. 2015. Mental Health Impacts. *In:* Levy, B. S. & Platz, J. (eds.) *Climate Change and Public Health.* New York: Oxford University Press.

Escobar, O., Morton, S., Lightbody, R. & Seditas, K. 2017. *Hard to Reach or Easy to Ignore.* Edinburgh: What Works Scotland.

Fals-Borda, O. 1999. *The Origins and Challenges of Participatory Action Research.* Amherst, MA: University of Massachusetts at Amherst.

Frank, A. 1995. *The Wounded Storyteller: Body, Illness, and Ethics.* Chicago, IL: University of Chicago Press.

Frank, A. 2010. *Letting Stories Breathe: A Socio-Narratology.* Chicago, IL: University of Chicago Press.

Frohmann, L. 2005. The framing safety project. *Violence Against Women,* 11, 1396–1419.

Hague, G., Harvey, A. & Willis, K. 2012. *Understanding Adult Survivors of Domestic Violence in Childhood: Still Forgotten, Still Hurting.* London: Jessica Kingsley.

Heginworth, I. S. & Nash, G. (eds.) 2019. *Environmental Arts Therapy: The Wild Frontiers of the Heart.* London: Routledge.

Huss, E. 2013. *What We See and What We Say: Using Images in Research, Therapy, Empowerment, and Social Change.* London: Routledge.

John, E. & Taupin, B. 1983. *I'm Still Standing.* London: Rocket Music Ltd.

John, E. & Taupin, B. 1989. *Sacrifice.* London: Rocket Music Ltd.

Kalmanowitz, D. & Lloyd, B. 2004. Inside the Portable Studio: Art Therapy in the Former Yugoslavia 1994–2002. *In:* Kalmanowitz, D. & Lloyd, B. (eds.) *Art Therapy and Political Violence: With Art, Without Illusion.* London: Routledge.

Kalmanowitz, D. & Lloyd, B. 2011. Inside-Out Outside-In: Found Objects and Portable Studio. *In:* Levine, E. G. L. & Stephen, K. (eds.) *Art in Action: Expressive Arts Therapy and Social Change.* London: Jessica Kingsley Publishers.

Kaur-Ballagan, K., Gottfried, G. & Day, H. 2021. Attitudes towards immigration: Survey conducted on behalf of IMIX. Available: https://www.ipsos.com/sites/default/files/ct/news/documents/2021-01/attitudes-towards-immigration-imix-2021.pdf [Accessed 29/5/22].

Kelly, L. 1988. *Surviving Sexual Violence.* Cambridge: The Polity Press.

Lempert, L. B. 1996. Women's strategies for survival: developing agency in abusive relationships. *Journal of Family Violence,* 11, 269–290.

Lloyd, G. 1993. *The Man of Reason; 'Male' & 'Female' in Western Philosophy.* London: Routledge.

Lloyd, B., Press, N. & Usiskin, M. 2018. The Calais winds took our plans away: art therapy as shelter. *Journal of Applied Arts & Health,* 9, 171–184.

May, V. 2013. *Connecting Self to Society: Belonging in a Changing World.* Basingstoke: Palgrave.

McKenzie-Mohr, S. & Lafrance, M. N. 2011. Telling stories without the words: 'Tightrope talk' in women's accounts of coming to live well after rape or depression. *Feminism & Psychology,* 21, 49–73.

Mclaren, M. 2004. Foucault and Feminism: Power, Resistance, Freedom. *In:* Taylor, D. & Vintages, K. (eds.) *Feminism and the Final Foucault.* Urbana, IL: University of Illinois Press.

Murphy, A. 2012. *Violence and the Philosophical Imaginary.* New York: State University of New York Press.

Myers, M. 2010. "Walk with me, talk with me": the art of conversive wayfinding. *Visual Studies,* 25, 59–68.

Nixon, R. 2011. *Slow Violence and the Environmentalism of the Poor.* New York: Harvard University Press.

O'Neill, M. 2008. Transnational refugees: the transformative role of art? *Forum Qualitative Sozialforschung/Forum: Qualitative Social Research,* 9, 2. Available: https://doi.org/10.17169/fqs-9.2.403 [Accessed 29/5/22].

O'Neill, M. 2009. Making connections: ethno-mimesis, migration and diaspora *Psychoanalysis, Culture & Society,* 14, 289–302.

O'Neill, M. 2010. *Asylum, Migration and Community.* Bristol: The Polity Press.

O'Neill, M. & Hubbard, P. 2010. Walking, sensing, belonging: ethno-mimesis as performative praxis. *Visual Studies,* 25, 46–58.

Pink, S. 2004. *Home Truths: Gender, Domestic Objects and Everyday Life.* Oxford: Berg.

Pink, S. 2007a. *Doing Visual Ethnography.* London: Sage.

Pink, S. 2007b. Walking with video. *Visual Studies,* 22, 240–252.

Pink, S. 2009. *Doing Sensory Ethnography.* London: Sage.

Rose, G. 1993. *Feminism and Geography: The Limits of Geographical Knowledge.* Cambridge: The Polity Press.

Rust, M. 2020. *Towards an Ecopsychotherapy.* London: Confer Books.

Singh, J. 2018. *Unthinking Mastery: Dehumanism and Decolonial Entanglements.* New York: Duke University Press.

Sinha, I. 2007. *Animal's People.* New York: Simon and Schuster.

Stanczak, G. C. (ed.) 2007. *Visual Research Methods.* London: Sage Publications.

Stoetzler, M. & Yuval-Davis, N. 2002. Standpoint theory, situated knowledge and the situated imagination. *Feminist Theory,* 3, 315–333.

5 Climate crisis

This chapter synthesises key features and observations that have emerged in the proceeding chapters. Reference is made to the ideas presented in Chapter 2 emerging from ecotherapy, ecopsychology, and environmental art therapy. It brings together the concepts of crisis, belonging, and imagination, which have been examined theoretically and practically in Chapters 3 and 4. It has been identified elsewhere how the arts have a role to play in addressing climate change where it is combined with psychology and other disciplines, with an emphasis on positive adaption to the social implications of climate change, particularly the results of increasing levels of migration and how this is responded to politically (Whomsley, 2021). Art therapy can take its place amongst other art-based practices in meeting such an objective. With that in mind, in this chapter I provide examples of how a model of social action art therapy can be applied practically by other art therapists, within the context of responding to climate crisis in ways that help individuals and groups stay with the truth, adapt, and act in ways that will assist processes of mitigation and adaptation. To help illustrate the ideas presented in this chapter, outlines are provided of workshops conducted with different groups, within which art has been used to explore the emotional responses of knowledge about climate and ecological crisis, and to imagine future forms of mitigation and adaptation. Aspects of art therapy and arts-based research are used together in a way that can be considered to be examples of what social action art therapy looks like in practice. Three broad groups of people took part in the workshops: environmental activists, university staff and students, and people who access community spaces and activities. These groups do of course overlap.

Within the workshops conducted, what has been identified is that there are a wide range of feelings initially expressed in response to considering climate change and crisis. These include anger, despair, guilt, helplessness, and isolation. Working individually to start with, and then collectively, participants have used visual mediums, music, and movement to explore those feelings in more detail and to start to imagine

DOI: 10.4324/9781003142560-5

how communities or organisations might respond to the growing consequences of climate change. Emotionally, what often arises at the end of participation is a sense of not being so isolated, and of feelings being validated and normalised. Whilst hope for solutions that might mitigate the impact of climate change is present, there is more of an expression of ideas and feelings that can be read as offering potential ways of preparing for, and living with, the predicted consequences of climate change. These have been both tangible and intangible. For example, students wanting the public spaces of their university to become softer and greener in the sense of having more indoor plants, but also in the sense of being less corporate and more like a space that they felt belonged to them. Relating this to the themes that appear in Chapter 4, what is observable is the construction of transitional stories and visions of adaptation that incorporate aspects of belonging. What has also occasionally arisen is reference to ideas about solidarity with other parts of the world that are more immediately exposed to the effects of climate change, and a desire to work with those who hold different views about climate change; both of which indicate that the ideas about fairness and bridging are close to the surface of many people's thoughts about climate crisis. Some challenges of working this way are given – in particular, the ongoing challenge of translating what emerges from the different groups into impactful policy at local and institutional levels. Example workshop plans are supplied as an appendix.

Workshop 1: environmental activists

The first workshop to be planned and facilitated took place in August 2019. It was a direct response to the intensity of emotions I was observing not only in myself but also those people I was coming into contact with as part of large-scale non-violent direct actions orchestrated by *Extinction Rebellion* taking place in the United Kingdom at that time. It is important to identify at this point how much I was emotionally affected by my growing acceptance of the reality of the climate and ecological crisis. As the *Climate Psychology Alliance* (CPA) would phrase it, I was struggling to face uncomfortable truths and uncertain futures. The feelings I had then, and still do have to varying degrees, can be categorised as fear, grief, anger, and guilt. Loss of sleep and a growing inability to concentrate being the physical manifestation of those feelings. These are not uncommon feelings to have in response to climate crisis (Dodds, 2021). And whilst eco-anxiety and climate-anxiety are frequently applied terms used to describe such feelings, they are terms that have been critiqued for being too simplistic a way to frame a complex set of emotions and responses (Bednarek, 2019). They can too easily suggest, or be interpreted as, a problem that is for individuals alone to address, and that are easily cured. A more subtle understanding, which helps to normalise and rationalise the feelings without minimising them, can be found in the concepts of eco-empathy (Sharp and Hickman, 2019) and solastalgia (Albrecht, 2005). Eco-empathy closes the gap between the human and the other-than-human and embraces a fundamentally human need to care and offer stewardship. Solastalgia draws attention to the loss of a sense of belonging to an environment, and is especially pertinent given the earlier observations about migration and violence disrupting a sense of belonging and forming a major part of transitional journeys and stories.

As part of my attempt to make sense of what I was learning about climate crisis (sometimes re-learning after a long period of amnesia and distraction), and to respond in a way that would be helpful to those around me and beyond me, I arrived at the intuitive realisation that I could take ideas and methods used in other contexts – set out in Chapter 4 – and apply those to climate crisis. It was during this time that I encountered the work of Joanna Macy and Chris Johnstone (Macy and Johnstone, 2012). Macy is a long-standing activist and workshop leader who has been engaging with the issue of climate crisis and other major issues, such as the proliferation of nuclear weapons, for many decades. As such, she has developed insights and guidelines that are extremely helpful in maintaining a sense of what she terms 'active hope' over the sustained periods of time that activism requires. Active hope is the ability to maintain hope and act with courage in the face of suffering and injustice. The importance of staying with what is difficult whilst maintaining hope and courage is articulated in striking form where Macy and Johnstone state that 'of all the dangers we face, from climate change to nuclear wars, none is so great as the deadening of our response' (p. 18). Avoiding such a danger is far from being an easy process when much of society and culture is structured around rewarding *not* taking care (Weintrobe, 2021). It is to avoid the deadening of our responses and to remain caring that Macy frames her work as a form of reconnection: reconnection with nature, spirit, creativity, and community. The practices developed by Macy and Johnstone align more closely to a creative and expressive approach to the use of the arts than they do to a psychotherapeutic use. This is because they are more focused on the present and upon identifying actions. There is also a strong explicit focus upon the communal and systemic problems and responses to climate crisis, rather than only focussing on individual psychological responses. As earlier chapters have addressed, there is much to be gained when blending sociological and psychological perspectives within a therapeutic context, and a social action approach to art therapy does this. An additional point of reference and inspiration is the *Through the Door* (CPA, 2021) initiative developed and offered by the CPA within which people are helped to process their emotional responses to climate crisis. The CPA primarily adopts a social psychology approach to thinking about and responding to climate crisis, and whilst my familiarity with their work was not great when initially starting out on developing my own response, they have since become an essential ally. These influences, together with those practices of eco-therapy and environmental arts therapies introduced in Chapter 2, provided a solid foundation on which to build the work.

In addition to this theoretical foundation, an important point to note here is that the planning and delivery of the majority of the workshops described in this chapter were the product of working collaboratively. This included developing the ideas in an iterative way with fine artist, Lor Bird[1], and colleagues from the University of Derby, Dr Yoon Irons and Dr Gemma Collard-Stokes. Yoon specialises in the use of singing and music within health and social care (Irons et al., 2020; Irons and Hancox, 2021). Gemma specialises in the use of dance and movement (Collard-Stokes, 2020). Together, we have been able to introduce a good range of creative mediums into the delivery of this work. The workshops that we offer to environmental activists are founded on four key positions:

1   The workshop aims to hold emotions expressed about climate crisis using creative methods.
2   The focus will move from the individual to the group.
3   The focus will primarily be upon the present moment in time.
4   This is not a form of personal therapy, but it might be therapeutic and transformative.

The first position is self-explanatory, although the word 'hold,' might be rephrased as 'contain' or 'stay with' or 'pay attention to.' We use the word 'hold' as it expresses something of the physicality of what we are doing. Whatever the phrase, the importance of this first point is to normalise the feelings and reduce any sense of shame or isolation they may provoke in people. The second position expands upon this by explicitly moving towards collective and systemic responses – this is a position that most contemporary ecological and environmental movements adhere to. The third position, which refers to staying in the present moment, is adopted to keep a sense of safety and containment. This is deemed especially important given that groups generally meet only once. Scope to think about the future can appear, but in the context of working with activists we primarily stay in the present. The final position is also one that is designed to provide emotional safety for the group and, together with the staying in the present, is necessary, given the brief nature of the group's existence. We find that three hours is a sufficient amount of time to set aside for the work if the activities and discussions are allowed to move at a gentle pace. Most groups have consisted of between six and eight people. A small group and a slow-pace allows participants to work safely together. After introducing these positions and ourselves, we ask each person to introduce themselves, including what brought them to the workshop. It is at this point that people normally start to express the feelings they have been trying to make sense of or have been struggling to contain. These feelings can range from guilt about not doing enough as an individual, to anger towards governments, corporations, and media organisations for not doing enough at a systemic or policy level – or where they have deliberately delayed meaningful actions. Fear of the future is common, especially for those who are parents or grandparents. There can also be confusion expressed about what is the best response, and sometimes expressions of doubt about the ability to do anything meaningful given the scale of what is being faced. For activists especially, the tension between feeling compelled to act and doubt about the value of actions taken can be especially acute. Burnout and ambivalence are real dangers within activism (Chen and Gorski, 2015; Lertzman, 2015), so we are especially mindful of the expressions of these feelings. The very act of being able to voice these feelings and having them accepted in a group environment is itself a powerful experience that diminishes isolation and shame. In a similar way, *Extinction Rebellion* encourages a regenerative culture, recognising that sustained activism without self-care leads to burnout and the appearance of destructive inter-group dynamics; and whilst *Extinction Rebellion* can be critiqued for its initial lack of acknowledgment of existing indigenous and global communities of resistance and rebellion, its contribution to bringing the emotional components of responding to the climate crisis into focus is to be praised. Inviting participants to introduce their feelings about climate crisis addresses the second position early on (that the focus will move from the individual to the group) because it enables the appearance of common thoughts and feelings at the very start of the group.

Following these introductions, we move on to the first arts-based activity. This entails introducing the theme of paying attention to what is often overlooked and of giving space to what is small or taken for granted. This can be taken as a reference for how aspects of the natural environment and uncomfortable feelings are often overlooked or not valued. To help give a frame to this theme we share Figure 5.1 with the group and quote the words of 14th-century English anchorite Julian of Norwich:

> And in this he showed me a little thing, the quantity of a hazel nut, lying in the palm of my hand, as it seemed. And it was as round as any ball. I looked upon it with the eye of my understanding, and thought, 'What may this be?' And it was answered generally thus, 'It is all that is made.' I marvelled how it might last, for I thought

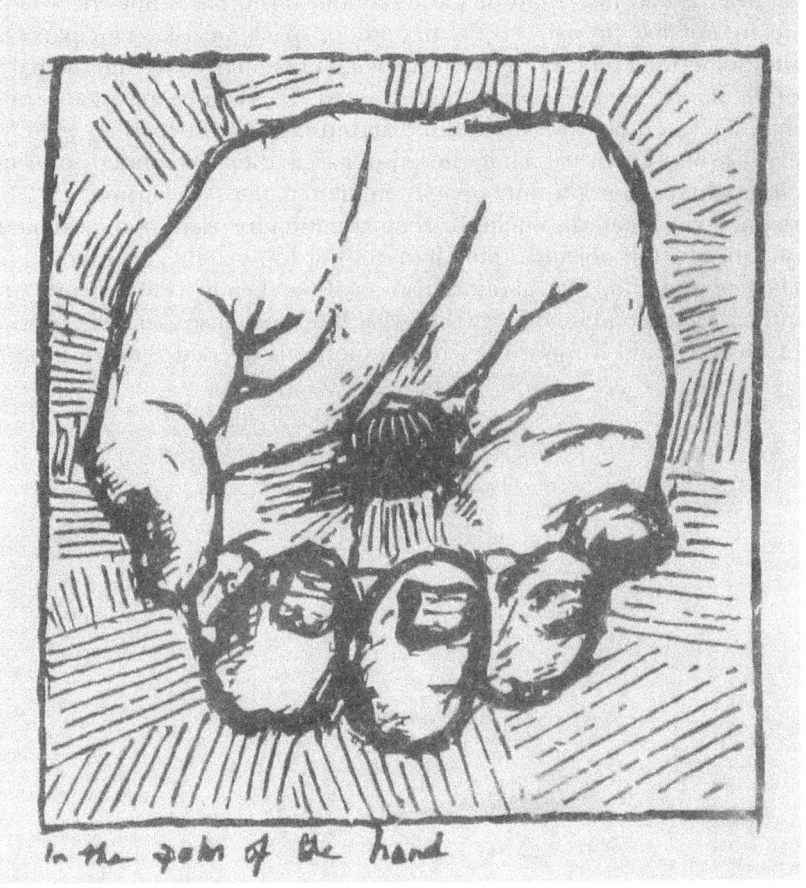

Figure 5.1 In the palm of the hand (Ink on paper by Jamie Bird)

it might suddenly have fallen to nothing for littleness. And I was answered in my understanding: It lasts and ever shall, for God loves it. And so have all things their beginning by the love of God. In this little thing I saw three properties. The first is that God made it. The second that God loves it. And the third, that God keeps it.

(John-Julian, 1991, p. 11)

We take care to couch this quotation as emerging from of a specific cultural and religious tradition, suggesting that participants might instead want to think of nature as being responsible for the making, loving, and keeping of what is small and precious. This quotation is just one of many that could be chosen; the purpose is to provide a poetic starting point. Participants are then guided to enter an outdoor green space, where we have access to such a space, to and look for some small natural object that could be gathered and taken back indoors. Where we are not able to easily access an outdoor space, we ask participants to find something on their person that is small enough to fit into the palm of the hand and is often taken for granted. This can be an organic or a manufactured object. We do not discriminate. It is surprising what we carry around with us! That chosen object is then responded to using either charcoal or graphite pencils on plain paper (see Figure 5.2). The restriction in materials helps to keep attention focused on the essential qualities of the object rather than getting too caught up in aesthetic choices and thoughts about artistic skill or beauty. Participants are guided to respond in any way they wish. This response can be figurative or abstract, and if more than one response is needed there is usually

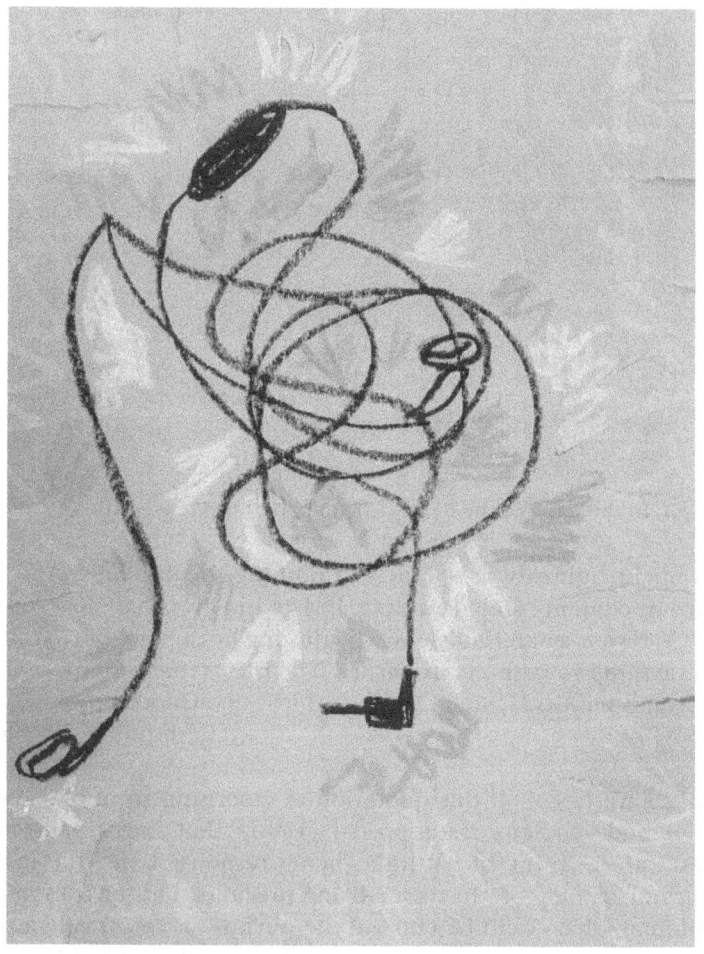

Figure 5.2 Response to first activity (Photo by Jamie Bird)

time to do that. Not only does this activity introduce the idea of paying attention to what is small, overlooked, or taken for granted, it also introduces a fundamental feature of most forms of art therapy and expressive therapies: that the process of creativity has equal, if not more, weight than the end product. We encourage a playful approach to creativity and to the materials used. After each person has a chance to introduce what they have made, and after a short comfort and refreshment break if needed, we move on to the second and main activity.

During the second activity we facilitate a more sustained use of creative activity. One such activity involves introducing participants to a wide selection of recycled packaging material. We both provide some ourselves and encourage participants to bring some of their own. Where we have moved workshops to an online format due to Covid-19 restrictions, participants providing their own recycled materials has proven to be helpful in allowing the work to continue. The use of recycled materials reflects several ideas: it follows on from the earlier theme of paying attention to what is overlooked; it embodies the act of reusing and recycling as an important component of climate change mitigation and adaptation; and it allows us to introduce the notion that what is human in origin is as natural a phenomenon as any other (Bookchin, 1989; Morton, 2009; Price, 2012). Can discarded packaging be as beautiful as a butterfly's wings? We introduce that last thought where a narrative emerges that suggests the expression of a sharp distinction between the human and the other-than-human, because a core concept within much ecological thinking is the closure of the conceptual gap between the human and the other-than-human. Participants are guided to use the recycled materials to create something that will express their thoughts and feelings about climate and ecological crisis, perhaps informed by what was shared in the group earlier. Where further guidance or inspiration is required we suggest that participants make use of the images they created within the first activity as a starting point. We very often do not provide glue, tape, or any other tools, so that participants have to be inventive with how they work with materials. As with the limiting of drawing materials to charcoal and graphite, this encourages being creative with what is provided. Figure 5.3 provides an example of what has been produced when working with recycled materials in this.

When individuals have had enough time to create what they need to create (30 to 40 minutes seems about right for this task), time is devoted to allow each person to verbalise their response to what they have created, and to explore the emotional and cognitive process involved in its making. The emergence of conversations within the group in response to the things made is encouraged where this allows a collective and shared understanding to appear. This collective approach links directly to the second position introduced above, of moving the focus

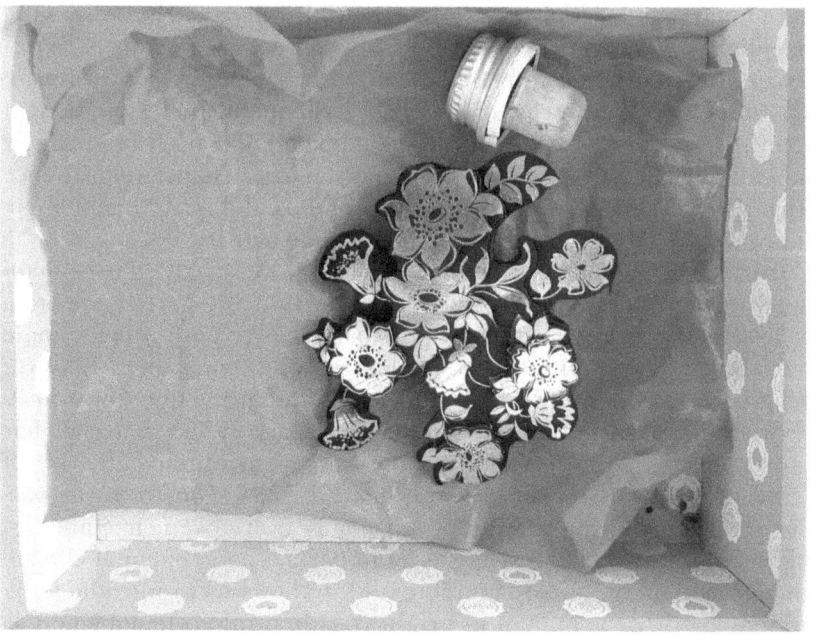

Figure 5.3 Using recycled materials (Photo by Jamie Bird)

from the individual to the group. It is also an essential component of working with the range of sometimes overwhelming feelings that arise in response to climate crisis, acknowledging that they are better accommodated and processed collectively. Just as the physical manifestations of climate change, and any meaningful mitigations and adaptations, are large in scale and so transcend individual responsibility and accountability, so too with the emotional manifestations, mitigations, and adaptations. This collective approach is further facilitated by asking participants to bring their own creations together to form a group response that reflects what has been shared. Because glue and tape has not been used, the reforming and interweaving of individual pieces into something collective can happen in a very fluid way. Figure 5.4 shows an example of this merging together of individual response to form a single collective response.

What we have observed is that where activists can come together in this way, they can find comfort in a shared acknowledgement of how difficult it can be to maintain whatever form their activism takes when there is so much to feel grief, despair, and guilt about. The creative component allows for the safe appearance and expression of such feelings, as well as bringing a playful component to the processing of those feelings. That this happens collectively enhances the power of acknowledging those feelings. Where activist participants are known to each

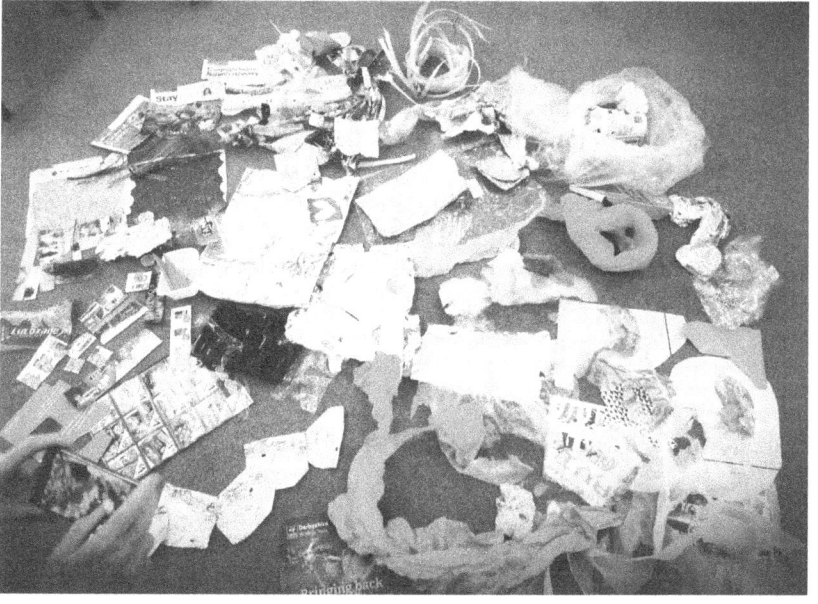

Figure 5.4 Collective response (Photo by Jamie Bird)

other, this can help to strengthen their ability to provide emotional support for one another at difficult moments, which in turn enables them to continue to be effective activists. What underpins the value of this aspect of the work is the notion of witnessing. Witnessing is a central component of both art therapy (Leahmonth, 1994), and to research that has an emancipatory intention. It points to the simple power of having stories and feelings seen and heard without prejudice, and to the act of witnessing being an ethical imperative within a just society (Levinas, 1999). From an ecological perspective, witnessing extends to how the experience of the other-than-human is manifested within the human, and how the other-than-human communicates itself to the human. What is the weather communicating? What are the trees saying? How do these appear within our thoughts, feelings, and stories? Responding to those questions requires a profound shift in perspective that runs counter to the dominance of human rationality over all other ways of knowing within modernity.

As these interactions with activists have progressed, we have, where this is relevant to what is being explored in the group, been able to bring to the discussion attention to the social justice elements of climate crisis. We have also observed social justice elements appear spontaneously within the topics explored and discussed within the groups. This growing inclusion of social justice as a component of climate crisis, as we have observed it, reflects the growing acknowledgement within those environmental movements based within the United Kingdom of the intimate and inescapable connection between different forms of injustice and exploitation. This reflects a broader shift in the United Kingdom, where, following the Black Lives Matter protests of 2019, anti-racism and de-colonialism are more explicitly expressed within political discourse and action. If viewed from the perspective of social action and social justice art therapy, the workshops, in addition to providing a space within which to have difficult feelings witnessed and honoured, provide useful psychological tools to activists to aid them in their active resistance to the damage done to the climate, the environment, and people. The primary tool is the one that enables individual participants to observe and acknowledge the collective nature of feelings about climate crisis.

Workshop 2: university staff and students

Building on the foundations of the work done with activists, the second group of people we have worked with are those people who are situated within university communities. This includes academics, support staff (ensuring the inclusion of an invitation to sub-contracted support staff), and students. We approach the notion of the university as being a whole unit, within which there are different and competing objectives and agendas that need to work together in order to identify options that are available to the institution in its response to climate crisis. The position taken in the workshop with activists that states: *the focus will primarily be upon the present moment in time,* now becomes: *the focus will move from being in the present to identifying imagined futures.* This shift in focus is informed by the research conducted with people who have experienced domestic violence and abuse outlined in Chapter 4, where the imagined future plays an important element in how stories of transition are constructed. It is also informed by our understanding of the importance, from the perspective of direct democracy and social justice, of ensuring that all opinions and voices are given attention within the decision-making process enacted by institutions. Whilst we are not able to guarantee that those ultimately making decisions will listen to those voices, we are working on ways to amplify them and make them harder to ignore. This process of amplification is aided by the production of artistic expressions, but still requires a great deal of effort in terms of generating interest within decision-making networks and forums if meaningful and long-term impact is to be achieved. At this point, that part of the process is still being formulated.

As with the workshops conducted with activists, we start with introductions that allow participants to express verbally whatever it is that currently pre-occupies them about the climate crisis. And like activists, members of the university community express a range of feelings such as confusion, anger, fear, and guilt. What varies is that the involvement in direct activism is often lesser within the university community, even if the desire to take action is just as strong. The idea of thinking together about how the university, as a community, might respond to climate crisis in terms of mitigation and transition is introduced early on to help give the group an overall focus. The first creative element sometimes follows the format of that used with activists, where attention is taken to that which is small or overlooked. This is a very transferable activity that most people can engage with and that helps to set the scene for thinking about aspects of ecology and climate crisis in a creative and playful way. The second part the workshop also follows a similar pattern, where participants are asked to make use of recycled materials to express their thoughts and feelings about climate crisis held at that time. We restate the focus upon the imagined future, suggesting that this might be something that participants hold in mind when working creatively with materials. After allowing sufficient time to pass, participants are guided towards bringing individual pieces together to create a larger collective piece.

As an alternative activity, when dancer Gemma Collard-Stokes co-facilitates the workshop, we use movement-based activities. For example, Gemma gives each participant an ice cube that they are invited to interact with as it slowly melts at room temperature. Participants are invited to respond to and document the slowly melting ice cube through any medium they have access to, including movement, art materials, written and spoken words, photography, or video made with smartphones. The invitation asks them to take responsibility for the life of an object and suggests that there are no limits to how they live out that time together. The point is that they pay attention to the moment-by-moment changes in state; the state of the melting ice cube and their own state from their position of responsibility and care. They are asked to consider how it makes a claim for its own agency and what their role is in that. The melting and shifting form of the ice cube is useful for encouraging a sense of the body and of a bodily relation to the object held; to consider how it feels to touch, hold, be marked by water and temperature, taste, smell; to notice and move in response to the ice cube's fleeting life.

Gemma has also asked participants, working as individuals and working in pairs or small groups, to translate their felt responses to various words associated with climate crisis into movement. Participants are asked initially to write one- or two-word response to listening to a poem, with the work of John Clare being helpful here. The words from this are often positive, uplifting, and optimistic. They then set that word aside. The group then looks at associations for these commonly used words in the media and respond to them through physical and embodied actions. Words that appear within the media include 'emergency,' 'catastrophe,' 'threat,' 'annihilation,' and 'extinction'; each of which have very evocative connotations. To this list can also be added the word 'crisis'! There is the potential appearance of quite violent or intense movements. Gemma then asks participants to go back to the words they had following the poem reading and repurpose the movement they created to embody one of these words instead. The meaning behind this activity is to consider how the words used to describe climate change (where 'change' too easily softens the impact of what is happening) can trigger strong emotional responses that find expression physically as well as mentally. The danger being that strong emotional responses, which are not fully or consciously processed, become blockers to hope and to action, and to the appearance of apathy as a way of creating emotional safety in the face of despair (Lertzman, 2015). The workshops are safe and containing spaces within which to express and acknowledge those feelings. In response to the words provided, participants are encouraged to create movements, one for each word. To help participants engage with this activity, Gemma provides suggestions for the kinds of movements that could be used. Participants might respond mimetically, where representation of the word is achieved through use of the whole body. They might respond sonically, exploring how saying the word in different ways creates different vibrations, rhythms, and tones that can inspire the body to move to the sound being made. If responding conceptually, they move to express what is being suggested by the word (associations, memories, ideas that come up for the participant as they consider the word and its bigger picture). Or, they can respond metaphorically, which can be very helpful in inspiring movement or encouraging movement in different ways: 'Imagine your spine is a winding river. Your feet are the roots of a tree. Your skull is a floating balloon.' Gemma models these ways of working to offer visual examples with her own body. She might also add in other ideas to help move things along, asking 'Can you move this action through the space? Can you work on an animal level? Can you make your actions move from big to small? Can you reverse your actions?' This is helpful for those people not used to working with the body and so they have more material to work with.

The final component of the workshop involves the group being asked to consider, in a collective way, how their university can respond to climate crisis. The suggestion is made that it can be helpful to focus both upon shorter- and longer-term responses (one year to ten years perhaps) and to consider both acts of mitigation and adaptation. The group is encouraged to arrive at a set of statements that can be fed into university forums responsible for environmental responses. Some of these statements reflect very concrete action the university can take, such as switching off lights and screens overnight, or introducing a zero-waste shop on campus. Others reflect more structural changes: identifying environmental leaders within staff and students; the university to act as a role model and to question its corporate responsibility. Whilst others communicate a prevailing sense of disconnection between participants and the university as an institution, alongside a strong desire to acquire a greater sense of belonging to the university; thus, a request to make communal spaces within the university softer, greener, less corporate, and sterile, and giving greater ownership of the spaces to students to decide on how they should look and work. The idea that the university should re-wild its green spaces emerges often as a suggestion. One suggestion has been that there should be less focus on financial growth within higher education. Whilst the main focus is upon collective responses, individuals are also invited to say what they will individually take away from this workshop and how they might translate that into action.

Workshop 3: community groups

The third set of workshops that we have developed are those that seek to work with communities that are traditionally less likely to appear as engaged with environmental issues from a mainstream perspective. What is meant by this is that public expressions of concern about the environment are often framed as being exclusively for white, metropolitan, and middle-class people (a critique that is frequently used by deniers and delayers as a way of minimising those concerns), whereas the reality is that concern for the environment is be felt just as keenly by indigenous people, people of colour, and by people of many different social and cultural backgrounds. It is activists from the global south who are most likely to lose their lives campaigning against environmental degradation. Many environmental NGOs and activist groups are responding to criticisms of being too narrow in who they represent, and are working hard to broaden their representation. And groups such as the *Institute for Tribal Environmental Professionals*[2], United States; the *Black Environment Network*[3], United Kingdom; and the *Islamic Foundation for Ecology and Environmental Sciences*[4], United Kingdom, demonstrate that concern for the environment is not the preserve of one group of people.

These workshops align well with the principles of social action art therapy. They also build upon the findings to emerge from the research presented in Chapter 4 that is concerned with imagination, belonging, and transitional journeys, as they pertain to refuge, asylum, and domestic abuse. The objective has been to work with community groups, using social action art therapy along with arts-based research methods to provide a way for people to explore their emotional understanding of climate change, how they imagine it will impact upon their families and their communities in the future, and what they imagine future community responses might look like. We are interested in understanding how imagination and a sense of belonging can contribute to the ways in which communities transition and adapt to an uncertain future. We aim to produce knowledge of imagined community responses to issues related to climate change that can contribute to the development of plans that local and regional councils and authorities are putting in place to manage adaptations to climate change. We also aim to provide an experience of creative methods that can be used by communities to sustain their resilience in the face of changes that emerge because of climate change, and to help them to transition and adapt to those changes. In developing this aspect of the work, we have become increasingly focused on the need to engage with diverse communities. As Rosemary Randall writes, '[w]e need to emphasize creativity and involvement in developing scenarios and solutions. We need to reject one-size-fits-all scenarios. We need to listen to and involve diverse communities who will have very different priorities and responses' (Randall, 2009). Diverse, in this context, means those peoples and communities that would not normally appear within discussion and consultation about environmental measures. As noted above, concern for the environment and climate change is not the preserve of one group of people, but the way in which power and representation works within political discourse and subsequent decision-making, means that some groups have a more dominant position than others, or are harder to ignore (Escobar et al., 2017). We acknowledge that the idea of community is complex and that no community is a static or homogenous entity. The work with refugees described in Chapter 4 clearly shows how communities are both fluid and hybrid. What does this mean in the United Kingdom in terms of who is ignored and not fully represented? It means black, indigenous, and people of colour. It means people from the Gypsy, Roma, and Traveller community. It means working-class communities. It means people with disabilities. An individual might belong to more than one of those groups. Reflective of the complex and organic nature of community, these workshops are in a state of development as we work to build relationships with the assistance of existing networks held by faith groups and community arts groups. The development of this work is slow because it needs to be conducted with humility, care, and attention. Like the work conducted within a university context, how the workshops interface with decision makers is an important part of the process and how we hope to demonstrate practical impact in the future. But, developing impact requires time and effort to bring to fruition, and so is still ongoing at this stage of development.

Where we have been able to implement some of these ideas, we have observed similar responses to those that emerge within the workshops for activists and for university staff and students. There has been concern expressed for the environment and for the ways in which climate change is appearing, along with the attendant feelings of fear, guilt, anxiety, and doubt that we have seen appear elsewhere. The workshops we have conducted at a community level have incorporated elements of the other workshops. Starting the group by paying attention to natural or manufactured objects that are small or delicate, again helps to set the tone and pace of the workshop. The use of recycled packaging materials to create larger pieces and to facilitate collaboration between participants works just as well in this context as it does in others. At this point, we have worked with young people who make use of a community café that is situated within an urban park, which is itself located in a city neighbourhood with a long history of housing newly arrived individuals and families from many parts of the world. There are established communities of Pakistani and Indian descent, a large number of people from Eastern Europe who have settled in the United Kingdom from the 1940s onwards, as well as families and individuals classed as asylum seekers who might only be temporarily living in the area but who may also choose to remain if and when granted permanent residency. The latter group reflects shifting geo-conflict conflicts; thus, the presence of people from Bosnia and Herzegovina, the Democratic Republic of Congo, the Kurdistan Region, Syria, and Libya. We have also worked with groups of people who make use of a community arts organisation, *Artcore*[5], who are a creative provider of activities to diverse communities, many of whom are at the margins of society. They work with various groups including older people, people with learning difficulties, physical and mental health problems, young people, and families. They aim to provide a creative platform of expression supporting and strengthening local networks and helping people to live a full and varied life.

When working with younger people within the community café space there was an opportunity for us to have conversations with young people, and any adults who accompanied them, about their understandings and responses to climate change, using creativity as an instigator for those discussions. What we delivered ran over two days, as part of a wider event that sought to engage the public in science. This took place just a week before the first UK-wide lockdown in response to Covid-19 in March 2020, so most conversations also included reference to what was most pressing at that moment in time. And perhaps the sense of uncertainty and dread experienced then about Covid-19 parallels something of the how the anticipation of climate change works for those who have not experienced its most extreme forms. With the café being attached to a park, we could use the outdoor space for some activities where needed. One way in which this developed was where, in response to the discussion within the group, we went litter picking with a small group of young people, who were mostly of Czech Republic and Romany origin. There was surprise expressed at the amount of litter and of how the harder you look, the more you see. This nicely links to how we ask people to pay attention to what might ordinarily be overlooked or discarded at the start of many workshops, with this itself being a metaphor for paying careful attention to emotions and feelings that might be overlooked. A theme that appeared when talking to the young people from Eastern Europe, was that whilst concern about climate change was not expressed as a priority, the sense of a strong connection to nature was evident. An adult from the Roma community stated how living sustainably was a normal way of life when resources and space are limited, and that a connection to nature is of great importance to the Roma community. Whilst no conclusion should be drawn from these brief exchanges, they do reveal that if the conversation is allowed to move beyond the confines of climate change, other pertinent themes will emerge. When using creative activities, which was again focused on the use of recycled materials, those young people who participated were able to express something of their thoughts and feelings about climate change visually. Figure 5.5 provides one example of this, and it shows beautifully how

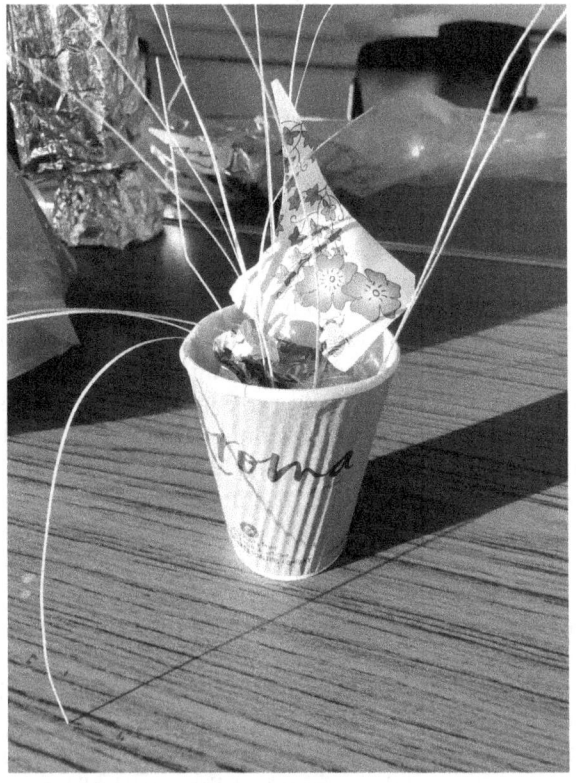

Figure 5.5 Aroma (Photo by Jamie Bird)

an appreciation for natural forms can be expressed using manufactured materials.

An example of where we have used these community-focused practices in a more open-ended way is to offer a space for children to use the materials we supply to make objects within a natural space as part of a public engagement event timed to coincide with COP26. As well as the inherent value of children being given the chance to be playful and creative in a natural space, a useful outcome of this work was where those adults who accompanied the children engaged with us in conversation about their own response to climate change. This included how they were concerned about the mental health of children and what sort of future they might have. These sorts of conversations present an opportunity both to listen to the concerns, and to direct parents and carers to those resources that exist to support them in providing good emotional support for children and young people who are concerned about climate crisis. This includes resources provided by the CPA to help parents and carers in that task. What this event shows, and the ones conducted within the community café, is that often the use of creativity is a helpful way of starting conversations around the issue of climate change. Conversations that can help to explore and normalise the associated feelings. Conversations that can help to make rational sense of information. Conversations that might be an instigator of further action. This meets the call to make such conversations a regular occurrence (Corner and Clarke, 2018; Sharp and Hickman, 2019), acknowledging that they have a crucial part to play within the broad range of direct, indirect, individual, and collective actions that are needed in response to climate crisis. As the climate crisis deepens and expands there will be a greater and greater need to have these kinds of conversations; to make them a common and spontaneous occurrence.

Transitional stories: part 2

How then do the themes that can be identified as forming transitional stories within experiences of migration and domestic violence, explored in Chapter 4, appear within the work described here that addresses climate crisis? As a reminder, those themes are *escape and harmony, relationships and social support,* and *agency and resistance.* And where does belonging and adaptation appear? Within the workshops with activists, there is a very explicit addressing of those feelings that, if not attended to, get in the way of the free and rational expression of political agency and resistance. In those same groups, where participants are often known to each other, the work can help to strengthen and deepen existing relationships and networks of social support. That strengthening can also be framed as an important contributor to the maintenance of a sense of belonging, which is so important to keeping activist groups going over the long term. The work with university students and staff, with its strong focus upon identifying imagined futures fits well with that aspect of transitional stories that is concerned with how the future might appear. It also allows for the emergence of thoughts about adaptation to climate change. This includes a consideration of how practices from the past might be reprised and brought into the future. What is also observed is how staff and students would want to see the university as a place that was in harmony with the organic and the natural. This expresses a very place-based response to the question of what the future might look like, and would also appear to aid a sense of participants belonging to the university and of the university belonging to them. That desire for belonging also seems to be expressed in wanting to see more accountability and leadership within the university in relation to its strategy and actions to address the climate crisis. For work with the wider community, adaptation and agency are the explicit focus from our perspective, where we aim to think about the future and generate ideas that can contribute to public policy, but just as important, and more frequently expressed by participants, is the desire for a sense of harmony and for some sense of belonging to place. Because the work with communities is in its early phase, it is difficult to say precisely how a consideration for the future, or other aspects of transitional stories, might emerge – if at all. It may be that focusing on the present is of more value for some groups than it is for others and that addressing the imagined future is for later on, requiring a more sustained level of commitment to working with those communities less represented within political decision-making processes. The suggestion that where people are unemployed, working on low incomes, or are in precarious housing and employment, or where people are made vulnerable by a sexist or racist society, there is little scope for them to think about or to act upon a changing climate, needs testing and challenging (Philo and Happer, 2013). As the effects of climate change become more apparent and immediate within everyday life, for those that have so far not had to address its effects, it will become more of an immediate concern, but that work needs to start now. And if the formula, as proposed by social ecology, that the crisis of ecological collapse can *only* be addressed by first tackling those social hierarchies rendered manifest within social injustices (Price, 2012), is taken at all seriously, then that work is essential.

The notion of the transitional story is just one way of framing how people might think and feel about their relationship to climate crisis, and there is scope for further work to be done on how this might relate to thoughts about adaptation to climate change. It does though offer a useful way of making some sense of both the feelings associated with fear, loss, and the disruption to a sense of self, place, and belonging, and of how the future might be imagined in a way that strengthens or recovers a sense of belonging. There are parallels that can be drawn between these transitional stories and the way in which individuals and communities express loss and belonging following experiences of political and domestic violence, even though for the people and groups we have worked with, the violence of climate change is most often either experienced in a vicarious or secondary way, or is in the shape of violence that is anticipated and dreaded. The strongest parallel between what has been expressed in the work presented here, when considering responses to climate crisis, and other forms of transitional stories, is how the imagined future contains ways of being and acting that either already exist or are able to be recovered from the past. Especially pertinent is where there is reference to a greater sense of reusing materials and making domestic items and clothing last longer through mending and repair. Also pertinent is the reference to the formation of strong community bonds and the building of bridges between different communities. How much of either of those are new solutions, or have existed in the past, is up for debate given that the past is as much an act of imagination as it is an act of remembering. The notion that indigenous ecological knowledge can somehow be recovered and repurposed by people who have long ago moved away from the land into towns and cities is perhaps far-fetched, but there is a surprising amount of such knowledge lying just below the surface of modernity, waiting to be unearthed. The important point is that the story contains links between the past and future in a way that provides a sense of resilience and of hope.

Challenges

Having introduced the different ways in which aspects of art therapy and arts-based research can be used in ways that contribute to the work of helping individuals and groups to make emotional sense of the climate crisis and to prepare for an uncertain future, the question needs to be asked: *Does this provide an adequate example of the practical application of social action art therapy?* Recalling those definitions of social action therapy introduced in Chapter 2, it is possible to say that the work presented acknowledges that individuals do not exist in a social vacuum (Kaplan, 2005), do aim towards the formation of just and peaceful communities (Hocoy, 2007), and are examples of 'a participatory, collaborative process that emphasizes artmaking as a vehicle by which communities name and understand their realities, identify their needs and strengths, and transform their lives in ways that contribute to individual and collective well-being and social justice' (Golub, 2005, p. 17). Keeping in mind the most salient features of social justice art therapy (Talwar, 2019), in starting to work with a broader range of communities there is the beginning of an attempt to more explicitly address the intersections of race, class, gender, and disability, within how individuals and communities are impacted by, and respond to, climate crisis. Engaging with a wider range of communities is a requirement if the work is to fully meet the potential of contributing to the well-being of individuals and communities, and the expansion of social justice that social action art therapy offers. That engagement will come about through the forming of trusting relationships and this takes sustained time and exertion. Where more attention is also needed, in order to align the work more fully with both social action and social justice, is the need to embed the method within places, communities, and institutions, so that there is an opportunity to generate long-term and meaningful change. In particular, and as indicated a number of times above, there is much work to be done on translating what emerges from the workshops into forms of communication that have an impact upon the creation of policies and governance procedures at an institutional and governmental level. Making the work sustainable and impactful is what is truly needed if it is to contribute to a future that is more just.

As a final thought about potential challenges, during Covid-19 restrictions of 2020 and 2021, some the work had to be adapted to be delivered online. And whilst that version of delivery and participation is not dwelt on here, it is worth noting that it worked surprisingly well. Reflective silences that might normally appear when meeting in person were often lacking, but there was nevertheless good engagement with the ideas and the practices amongst the groups who took part in online versions of these workshops.

Summary

Transferring ideas and practices developed when employing arts-based research – that is itself informed by elements of art therapy – within the context of seeking to better understand refuge and asylum, and domestic violence and abuse, are here shown to have value in responding to climate crisis. The blending of research and therapy, where there is an equal emphasis upon elucidation, emancipation, and transformation, appears within how social action art therapy has been presented in earlier chapters. Social action art therapy also explicitly acknowledges and woks with the communal and political aspects of experience. It is this approach that underpins the work described here in this chapter. Given the strange nature of climate crisis – how it indiscriminately pervades space and time, at the same time as being experienced very differently, dependent upon existing hierarchies and inequalities – there is a need to develop ways of working with it that can take account of the intersection of the personal and the political. A social action approach to art therapy provides this dual focus, especially when it is enhanced by reference to social justice. What also makes social action art therapy appropriate in working with climate crisis is how it opens a space for considering imagined futures that are both personal and collective. Where more attention is required, it is the development of ways of translating what emerges within the work described here into practical actions at a collective level. This is not just about imagined technical solutions to climate change; it is also about actions that can make a difference to how people communicate with each other, make decisions together, and take care of themselves and their surroundings. This entails community organising and working collaboratively with those making political decisions or decisions about the management of organisations.

The suggestion has been made that alternative ways of being in community and in relationship with the other-than-human are available, where reference can be made to historical evidence of such alternatives; ones that entail different ways of thinking about the distribution of power and of decision-making, or different ways of thinking about property and land ownership. The recovery of those alternatives, the reformation of them in ways that are suitable for a new future, along with the creation of unique and new alternatives will require engaging the collective imagination of communities and societies. Social action art therapy can take its place alongside other techniques for bringing about such a process of engagement and action.

Notes

1 https://lorbird.wixsite.com/artbylorbird [accessed: 25/1/2022]
2 https://www7.nau.edu/itep/main/Home [accessed: 14/9/2021]
3 http://www.ben-network.org.uk/index.asp [accessed: 14/9/2021]
4 https://www.ifees.org.uk/about/about-ifees/ [accessed: 14/9/2021]
5 https://www.artcoreuk.com/ [accessed: 15/11/2021]

References

Albrecht, G. 2005. Solastalgia: a new concept in human health and identity. *Philosophy Activism Nature*, 3, 41–44.
Bednarek, S. 2019. 'This is an emergency' – proposals for a collective response to the climate crisis. *British Gestal Journal*, 28, 4–13.
Bookchin, M. 1989. *Remaking Society*. Montreal: Black Rose Books.
Chen, C. & Gorski, P. 2015. Burnout in social justice and human rights activists: symptoms, causes and implications. *Journal of Human Rights Practice*, 7, 366–390.
Collard-Stokes, G. 2020. Recreational burlesque and the aging female body: challenging perceptions. *Journal of Women & Aging*, 34(2): 155–169.
Corner, A. & Clarke, J. 2018. *Talking Climate: From Research to Practice in Public Engagement*. Basingstoke: Palgrave Macmillan.

CPA. 2021. *Through the door: A therapeutic practice for the commons.* Climate Psychology Alliance [Online]. Available: https://www.climatepsychologyalliance. org/events/307-through-the-window [Accessed 09/08/21].

Dodds, J. 2021. The psychology of climate anxiety. *BJPsych Bulletin,* 45, 222–226.

Escobar, O., Morton, S., Lightbody, R. & Seditas, K. 2017. *Hard to Reach or Easy to Ignore.* Edinburgh: What Works Scotland.

Golub, D. 2005. Social action art therapy. *Art Therapy,* 22, 17–23.

Hocoy, D. 2007. Art Therapy as a Tool for Social Change: A Conceptual Model. *In:* Kaplan, F. (ed.) *Art Therapy and Social Action.* London: Jessica Kingsley Publishers.

Irons, J. Y., Garip, G., Cross, A. J., Sheffield, D. & Bird, J. 2020. An integrative systematic review of creative arts interventions for older informal caregivers of people with neurological conditions. *PLoS One,* 15, e0243461.

Irons, J. Y. & Hancox, G. 2021. *Singing.* West Yorkshire: Emerald Publishing.

John-Julian, O. J. N. 1991. *A Lesson of Love: The Revelations of Julian of Norwich.* London: Darton, Longman & Todd.

Kaplan, F. F. 2005. What is social action art therapy? *Art Therapy,* 22, 2.

Leahmonth, M. 1994. Witness and witnessing in art therapy. *Inscape. Journal of the British Association of Art Therapists,* 1, 19–22.

Lertzman, R. 2015. *Environmental Melancholia.* London: Routledge.

Levinas, E. 1999. *Alterity and Transcendence.* London: Columbia University Press.

Macy, J. & Johnstone, C. 2012. *Active Hope: How to Face the Mess We're in Without Going Crazy.* Novato, CA: New World Library.

Morton, T. 2009. *Ecology Without Nature: Rethinking Environmental Aesthetic.* Cambridge, MA: Harvard University Press.

Philo, G. & Happer, C. 2013. *Communicating Climate Change and Energy Security: New Methods in Understanding Audiences.* New York: Routledge.

Price, A. 2012. *Recovering Bookchin: Social Ecology and the Crises of Our Time.* Norway: New Compass Press.

Randall, R. 2009. Loss and climate change: the cost of parallel narratives. *Eco-Psychology,* 1, 118–129.

Sharp, V. & Hickman, C. (2019) Eco-anxiety, eco-despair, eco-depression, eco-grief? Or maybe ... eco-empathy?, *Climate Crisis Conversations* [Podcast]. 13/10/19. Available online: https://www.climatepsychologyalliance.org/~cpa/podcasts/402-podcast-eco-anxiety-eco-despair-eco-depression-eco-grief-or-maybe-eco-empathy [Accessed 10/02/22].

Talwar, S. 2019. *Art Therapy for Social Justice: Radical Intersections.* London: Routledge.

Weintrobe, S. 2021. *Psychological Roots of the Climate Crisis: Neoliberal Exceptionalism and the Culture of Uncare.* New York: Bloomsbury.

Whomsley, S. R. C. 2021. Five roles for psychologists in addressing climate change, and how they are informed by responses to the COVID-19 outbreak. *European Psychologist,* 26, 241–248.

6 Conclusion

An argument was put forward at the start of this book that this time in history presents a unique set of circumstances and intersecting crises that are manifesting themselves on a global scale. Within that argument, climate change is presented as the most pressing contemporary crisis, which in turn is emblematic of structural and philosophical contradictions that sit at the centre of modernity. It has also been strongly argued that climatic and ecological crises cannot be disentangled, or responded to separately, from the many forms of social crises that coexist with climate crisis. Writing this book, my own expanded appreciation of the weight of that argument mirrors how the wider environmental and climate action movement – in the United Kingdom at least, learning both from the United States and from histories of resistance outside of the global north – has embraced the intersections of environmental injustices and social injustices. Art therapy has a history of challenging injustices and the status quo, where it has confronted the medicalised response to psychological distress and offered alternative and complementary responses to medication or incarceration. It is prescient then to make links between how art therapy responds and reacts to different forms of social injustices, and to how the arts might be used to form transitional stories that help to make sense of, and gain agency, over those injustices. Existing models of social action and social justice approaches to art therapy show how art therapy can effectively work to address community distress in response to injustice. What is added to those approaches, in the ideas and practices presented here, is a focus on the role of violence within social injustice, and the way in which art therapy, through its ability to address collective trauma, and its ability to engage collective imagination, might assist in making a transition to a less violent and more just future. How that appears within responses to refuge, migration, and domestic violence and abuse is used as a foundation for then responding to climate crisis, where that crisis is taken to be another form of violence and injustice – albeit one that manifests at both a local level and a global level.

DOI: 10.4324/9781003142560-6

In considering the global scale of climate crisis, attention was drawn early on to how there is a requirement to be mindful of the power that certain words have of projecting a totalising or over-simplified meaning on what they are referring to, when a more nuanced and diverse understanding is required. Often, they assume that the reader is like the author. It is worth making this observation again, as the case I make for social action art therapy draws to a close. Words such as 'we,' 'humanity,' and 'nature' become problematic if not qualified by asking who or what is being referred to – or who or what is being excluded. This might appear pedantic and something that could just as easily be applied to many other words, but in the context of climate crisis, where social injustices are taken as coexisting and contingent crises, failure to highlight or contextualise those words that do not explicitly take account of difference and diversity is potentially detrimental to the objective of addressing those crises and the injustices. The same caution is necessary when considering the very use of the word 'crisis' and how that word can be co-opted to justify draconian and exclusionary actions and laws. A careful balance is also needed when using terms like 'climate crisis': to communicate the perilous state of the climate and of how, over the next decade, critical choices must be made about what sort of future societies are desired, at the same time as not wanting to trigger states of political and psychological panic that can lead to withdrawal, disavowal, or the further entrenching of racist and other exclusionary positions.

How communicating about climate crisis is complex and fraught, especially when applying the formula that there can be no meaningful response to climate crisis without equally responding to social injustice, is further illustrated by the range of ways in which ecological thought and action can been articulated. Amongst the many and varied ecologies available, four have been presented that I believe best serve the purpose of forming a social action art therapy response to climate crisis. Deep ecology, dark ecology, social ecology, and traditional ecological knowledge have been chosen because of their mix of psychological, sociological, and political positions. Deep ecology, dark ecology, and traditional ecological knowledge each bring a recognition of the power of the mythic and the poetic, whilst social ecology makes a very clear case for the need to take account of the appearance of power and hierarchy within human societies and within how those societies engage with the other-than-human. From the perspective of anti-racist and decolonial thought and practice within art therapy, it is traditional and indigenous ecological knowledge that offers a useful alternative to those psychologies that are primarily modern and western in origin and which inform so much of art therapy. Taken together, these ecologies seek to imagine a relationship between the human and the other-than-human that is based on respect for diversity, humility, and reciprocity. And, to a greater or lesser extent, they each extend those same qualities to how they imagine humans relating to each other. This conception of relationships within and between the human and the other-than-human differs from how those same relationships are imagined within the dominant political and economic systems that flow from modernity – primarily, the capitalist version of modernity – centred as it is upon industry, productivity, and resource extraction. These ecologies, especially traditional ecological knowledge, also do much to de-centre the primacy of human knowledge and experience (What do the trees remember? What does the land know?), which is itself a major counterpoint to modernity's hierarchy of knowledge.

Modernity, as a frequently referenced philosophical and political project, has been presented here as both a system of contradictions that comes about through the purification and specialisation of knowledge, where nature and the human exist in separate vacuums (Latour, 1993); and, when co-opted by capitalism, as a failed attempt to bring about a world of material abundance through permanent technological progress. Modernity has also been presented as a system of thought that centres 'whiteness,' using violence and coercion as a way of dominating, controlling, and sending to the margins that which deviates from that 'whiteness' (Echeverría, 2019). 'Whiteness' being defined by Echeverria as an ethics of personal sacrifice in the service of capital, emanating from European Protestantism, that not only elevates its own world view above all others, but actively seeks to suppress, exclude, and eliminate all other world views through violent means. Vanessa Andreotti's image of modernity being a crumbling house (Andreotti et al., 2015; Andreotti et al., 2018), born out of, propped up by, and undermined by violence – including state-sanctioned racism and genocide – underscores how central violence is to the maintenance of modernity's domination. Crucial to thinking about violence in that context is to consider how violence appears in the form of physical and non-physical acts of coercion and control, and of how violence is both state-sanctioned and institutionalised. The violence that is addressed in this book is violence that primarily occurs at a society level and a state level, as well as being violence that manifests itself across generations. This includes domestic violence and abuse, which whilst manifesting within interpersonal relationships is born out of, and sanctioned by, societal norms around gender and power.

Andreotti's critique of modernity also includes a call to imagine alternatives to modernity and to capitalism. Such a call to imagine alternative futures is a theme that is returned to throughout this book. Imagination, as both an epistemology and as a creative process, helps to join together art therapy, arts-based research, and social action. They each use imagination as a way of making sense of the past and the present, and of envisioning the future. This includes imagining what belonging means when violence is ongoing – slow or otherwise (Nixon, 2011) – and what it means to belong in the aftermath of violence. The reasons for putting forward the case that imagination is a valid epistemology for approaching the past, the present, and the future – which can be complementary to reason – are that it provides a means of providing a bridge between the individual and the other, and between the mind and the body (Stoetzler and Yuval-Davis, 2002; Leavy, 2007). A case has been made that framing imagination as both an embodied and a situated process fits with an intersectional and feminist understanding of both social justice and political action, where there is an emphasis upon therapist and researcher reflexivity, and being curious about the other. Such situated and embodied imagination does though entail entering a place of vulnerability and ambiguity (Villa, 2011; Murphy, 2012). Art therapy and arts-based research methods that are informed by art therapy, along with the images that emerge from those (which have their own existence beyond that of the artist and informant), are well-placed to stay with and work with the appearance of vulnerability and ambiguity.

To recap: violence, as a manifestation of modernity, and how that violence disrupts community and belonging (who belongs and who does not), has been shown to appear within experiences of migration and refuge, and experiences of domestic violence and abuse. In both of those cases, the importance of the body, objects, and places has been shown to be important in how people communicate their experiences. Art therapy and arts-based research methods provide a means of accessing that physicality in ways that are sensitive to the poetic, the irrational, and the metaphoric, as well as being attentive to the contextual and situated nature of experience and knowledge. A vital similarity between experiences of migration and refuge, and domestic violence and abuse, in addition to violence and belonging is how creativity and imagination can be used to identify potential ways of transitioning towards different futures that are not defined by violence or by a lack of belonging. Instead, those futures are founded on belonging, relationship, and agency. The lessons from working in those contexts provides a rationale for transferring the theory and practice across to responding to manifestations of climate crisis at a both a personal, community, and social level.

Because of the emphasis placed upon the communal and social elements of experience, social action, and social justice, art therapy presents a pertinent way of framing the response to all three of the contexts addressed in this book. Social action art therapy, as a model, is presented as folding the communal and the social into the psychological components of art therapy, recognising that individuals do not live in a historical, social, or political vacuum (Kaplan, 2005; Hocoy, 2007). A social justice approach to art therapy adds an explicit focus on the intersections of race, ethnicity, class, gender, sexuality, and disability to that model, whilst acknowledging the historical and political basis for existing forms of oppression (Talwar, 2019). I have proposed that around this model can be wrapped those ecological perspectives identified as having value to art therapy, so as to help move social action art therapy and social justice art therapy into a space that enables it to meet the challenges posed by climate crisis and the inescapable intersections it has with social and psychological crises. Weaving ecology into social action and social justice – and art therapy more generally – also helps to make art therapy practice more sensitive to those cultures and communities that have a tradition of not rigidly demarcating the boundary between the individual self, their community, and the landscape they are part of; with that tradition itself being a useful guide for other communities that are shaped by rigid conceptual boundaries between self, community, and nature. A vital challenge at this time is the need to imagine alternative futures and the need to identify ways of transitioning towards those futures – with both the journey and the destination being places of safety, inclusion, and care. How each individual and community imagines that future will be contingent upon their past and present material conditions? As stated repeatedly, the effects of climate crisis are not universally the same for all peoples. For some people, the present already means keeping alive valuable lessons from the past about how they overcame adversity and oppression. For others, it means recalling how to live an ecologically harmonious life. Whilst for other people, it will mean entering a time of great uncertainty, where their own collective memory is less of a useful resource for future use, and deep learning from others will be necessary.

The ideas and practices that I have presented do however pose a challenge, in terms of pushing at the boundaries of art therapy where there is an explicit merging of art therapy with arts-based research methods and with political and community activism. It is valid to ask: *Is this synthesis of approaches too broad for art therapy to contain and still be a safe and effective practice? Should art therapy confine itself to the intrapsychic and the interpersonal?* To the first question, the answer is that where the practice is developed and conducted from a place of both reflection and reflexivity, and where participants are fully aware of what it is they are engaged with, the work can be safe. Supervision and peer support being essential features of working safely. How effective the work is will depend on the stated goals. As identified in Chapter 5, translating the outputs from group encounters into something that has impact more widely, where political transformation is the goal, takes time and the building of relationships with people who hold power. This is not to take away from the very immediate positive impact engagement can have for participants. In fact, the appearance of self-reported beneficial effects, by participants taking part in arts-based research, has helped me to become comfortable with the notion that arts-based research can come to exhibit the features of art therapy, and to be transformative for participants. Remembering how the principles of emancipation sit at the centre of feminist thought, which in turn has informed the development of arts-based research practices (Leavy, 2007), provides additional support for adopting this position. The second question, about what art therapy should confine itself to, has been addressed throughout the arguments and examples put forward here. Extending art therapy out from the individual and the interpersonal, to embrace the communal, social, and the ecological, is appropriate where the causes of distress and injustice, and how those are manifested, is located at a collective level. Addressing individual and localised psychological distress is of course what many people want and need, and art therapy does that well. What is argued here, and within the broader field of social action and social justice approaches to art therapy, is that an expanded perspective is also required in many instances, and that this can complement other approaches to art therapy. There is a constant need to revisit the assumptions and foundations that support any approach and it is hoped that this book will contribute to the ongoing development and evolution of art therapy, be that with a focus on social action, social justice, or otherwise.

Where next? This is an uncertain but critical decade. The 2021 United Nations Climate Change Conference in Glasgow (COP26) delivered some hope, but only if promises and pledges are both strengthened and put into place will the best-case scenario of predicted global heating come into being. Every small incremental failure equals more devastation, more death, more extinction, and more unequal distribution of suffering. Rapid and large changes need to happen *this* decade for them to contribute to the goal of net-zero carbon emissions by 2050. If those changes are delayed for later decades, that 2050 target will not be met. However this plays out in the 2020s, there will be disruption and challenges: where changes are implemented new ways of living will need to be adapted to; where changes are not implemented there will be protest and resistance. In either case, anger and resentment will emerge. Violence can be predicted to arise in either scenario as people push back against change or inaction, and as national states work to maintain and exert control. And regardless of what change does or does not take place, an unpredictable climate is here now, with all the attendant problems and magnification of existing injustices that entails. The temptation for states to become more authoritarian and to make their borders stronger still will increase. The growing competition for natural resources will further inflame interstate tensions and conflict. All of that is pretty grim – to put it mildly – and one understandable response would be to close one's own emotional and cognitive borders in order to carry on with everyday life. There is though an alternative …

… to keep caring and to imagine that the future can be different; to be in relationship with each other and with the other-than-human that is full of gratitude, reciprocity, and humility; to imagine different ways of making political decisions; to come together and create communities that are robust and resilient enough to encompass diversity in whatever form that takes. Social action art therapy presents one way in which people can come together to address collectively the emotional components of climate crisis, and to imagine how they can individually and collectively make the transition to a future that is based on love and care.

References

Andreotti, V. O., Stein, S., Ahenakew, C. & Hunt, D. 2015. Mapping interpretations of decolonization in the context of higher education. *Decolonization: Indigeneity, Education & Society*, 4, 21–40.

Andreotti, V. O., Stein, S., Sutherland, A., Pashby, K., Susa, R. & Amsler, S. 2018. Mobilising different conversations about global justice in education: toward alternative futures in uncertain times. *Policy and Practice: A Development Education Review*, 26, 9–41.

Echeverría, B. 2019. *Modernity and "Whiteness"*. Cambridge: Polity.

Hocoy, D. 2007. Art Therapy as a Tool for Social Change: A Conceptual Model. *In:* Kaplan, F. (ed.) *Art Therapy and Social Action*. London: Jessica Kingsley Publishers.

Kaplan, F. F. 2005. What is social action art therapy? *Art Therapy*, 22, 2.

Latour, B. 1993. *We Have Never Been Modern*. New York: Harvester Wheatsheaf.

Leavy, P. 2007. Merging Feminist Principles and Art-Based Methodologies. *American Sociological Association Annual Conference*. New York.

Murphy, A. 2012. *Violence and the Philosophical Imaginary*. New York: State University of New York Press.

Nixon, R. 2011. *Slow Violence and the Environmentalism of the Poor*. Harvard: Harvard University Press.

Stoetzler, M. & Yuval-Davis, N. 2002. Standpoint theory, situated knowledge and the situated imagination. *Feminist Theory*, 3, 315–333.

Talwar, S. 2019. *Art Therapy for Social Justice: Radical Intersections*. London: Routledge.

Villa, P. 2011. Embodiment Is Always More: Intersectionality, Subjection and the Body. *In:* Lutz, H., Vivar, M. & Supik, L. (ed.) *Framing Intersectionality: Debates on a Multi-Faceted Concept in Gender Studies*. Farnham: Ashgate Publishing Limited.

Appendix: Example workshop plans

Workshop 1: environmental activists

Philosophies:

1 The workshop aims to hold emotions expressed about 'climate crisis' using creative methods.
2 The focus will primarily be upon the present moment in time.
3 The focus will move from the individual to the group.
4 This is not a form of personal therapy, but it might be therapeutic and transformative.

Timetable:

Framing
Outline the philosophies and objectives for this workshop. Participants will be encouraged not to talk over one another and to speak clearly to ensure that participants who are hearing impaired can fully engage with the workshop.

Start/introduction
A verbal introduction from each person that takes the form of responding to 'who you are?' and 'what brings you here?' Facilitators contribute to this.

House keeping
Cover health and safety and fire procedure and location of toilets and kitchen.

Ground rules
Identified and established by the group verbally, with notes taken. Draw attention to being able to 'step aside' if the work gets too much. Aim to complete these first elements within 30 minutes.

Task 1: Being present (60 minutes)
Introduce the words of *Julian of Norwich* and the 'In the palm of the hand' image with the themes of holding, gratitude, and seeing clearly made explicit by the facilitator. Participants are asked to select a small (and possibly overlooked object) from the garden/park (or on their person if outdoor space not available) which can fit in the palm of their hand, or from their person if it is raining. The object will be taken back to meeting room and drawn on recycled paper using charcoal and/or pencil for 45 minutes. There will be an opportunity to reflect on this task verbally within the group and is focused on the individual experience. It will last for 15 minutes.

Break: It is a chance to make journal notes if required and make a drink. Ten minutes given over to this.

Task 2: Group emotions (60 minutes)
Speak about the use of transient materials in a fluid way, and of how this links to the first task that focused on appreciating the small and the overlooked. Explain that there is no glue or tape, etc., as the aim is to create fluid images using just the materials people have chosen to bring with them. There are scissors for cutting and creating collage. Examples of what is possible using collage will be shown if required.

People are directed to first work alone and to respond to whatever feelings emerge when considering climate, environment, and ecology. All feelings are welcome – both light and shadow. After some time doing this individually, people will be directed to bring what they have created together with others to create a group montage/collage that contains everyone's responses but also builds on those individual responses. Here, there is the chance for people to reshape their image to take account of those around them. The group will be encouraged to do this non-verbally, reminding the group that there will be time to verbally respond later. When it feels like the group has worked long enough, they will be asked to verbally reflect on the task – to say what their individual responses were expressing and how those changed as they brought them into contact with other people's expressions. If anyone wishes to, they can make further changes to their element after the verbal responses are given.

Finally, photographs can be taken of what has been created before the group works together to dismantle that creation, reflecting on the transient and circular nature of what is made and expressed.

Close: 20 minutes
Individuals will be asked to say what they will take away from this workshop and how they might translate that into action. Participants will be able to browse through books that may be of benefit and a list of

hyperlinked online resources will be emailed out afterwards. Short feedback forms will be handed out for people to fill in before they leave which include evaluation of the workshop and the opportunity to make suggestions for further workshop ideas. We will verbally ask whether people would wish to be contacted again and whether they have suggestions for future workshops.

Workshop 2: university staff and students

Philosophies:

1 The workshop aims to hold emotions expressed about 'climate crisis' using creative methods.
2 The focus will primarily be upon the present moment in time, but will move to imagining the future.
3 The focus will move from the individual to the group.
4 This is not a form of personal therapy, but it might be therapeutic and transformative.

Timetable:

Framing: (5 minutes)
Outline the philosophies and objectives for this workshop. Participants will be asked not to talk over one another and to speak clearly to ensure participants who are who have hearing impairments can fully engage with the workshop.
    Cover health, safety, fire procedure, location of toilets, etc.

Ground rules: (5 minutes)
Identified and established by the group verbally, with notes taken. Draw attention to being able to 'step aside' if the work gets too much.

Introduction: (10 minutes)
A verbal introduction from each person that takes the form of responding to 'who you are?' and 'what brings you here?' Facilitators will contribute to this activity.

Task 1:
Introduce the words of Julian of Norwich and the 'In the palm of the hand' image with the themes of holding, gratitude, and seeing clearly made explicit. Participants are asked to select a small (and possibly overlooked object) from outside which can fit in the palm of their hand, or from their person if it is raining. The object will be taken back to the meeting room and drawn on recycled paper using charcoal and/or pencil for 45 minutes. There will be an opportunity to reflect on this task verbally within the group but is mainly focused on the individual experience.

Break: (15 minutes - if required)

Task 2: Body movement section (total of 90 minutes)

Activity one: Moving Body
Moving with increasing awareness and connection to ground/gravity/push/roll/energy moving through the body – individual responses leading to group moving through space exploring into and out of the floor.

Activity two: Moving Language

1 Read short poem by John Clare.
2 Participants asked to write a one-word emotional response to the poem on paper and set it aside.
3 Participants are asked to think of images/words/feelings they associate with climate crisis (emergency, catastrophe, threat, annihilation, extinction) and write on large paper.
4 Can participants pluck out or think of verbs for physical actions they connect with these words (seek, strike, batter, reach, crash, attack).
5 Working on their own, the participants are encouraged to choose four verbs and create four movements/actions to represent them using the whole body.
6 Participants then asked to repurpose the movements they have produced to embody the word they wrote down earlier – adapt the movement to serve the word/image/feeling you had following the poem.
7 Share with a partner and discuss.
8 Combine your work together and share with everyone – can we all explore together?

Activity three: An invitation to merge with landscape (outdoors)
Take a walk and find a place that invites your participation. Explore how you can become part of the landscape so that someone walking past might not even know you are there. For instance, enter a pile of leaves, lie between or under the crevices of foliage, or wrap your bod inside a shallow nook or around a tree branch. Be safe in your choice so that you can enjoy the sensations (10 minutes).

   Disappear into this place, becoming part of its skin and texture. See with its eyes, breathe with its breath (10 minutes).

   Separate yourself once again and pause in open attention. Draw or write about your experience. Consider whether release of identity expands awareness of self and other (10 minutes).

Activity four: An Invitation (indoors)

1 Each person is gifted a note and has time to read and digest this prior to the main activity.
2 They will then be gifted a material to work with (everyone receives the same material).
3 Each person is invited to respond to the material through movement/performed actions and then to follow this up with writing/drawing/moving, etc.
4 The note also includes an invitation to document their activity through image/gif/video/text if they so choose.

Future: 30 minutes
The group will be asked to consider, in a collective way, how the university can respond to climate crisis. It would be helpful to try to focus upon shorter- and longer-term responses (one year to ten years perhaps) and to consider both mitigation and adaptation. The group will be encouraged to arrive at a set of statements that can fed into university forums responsible for environmental sustainability.

Individuals will also be asked to say what they will individually take away from this workshop and how they might translate that into action.

Participants will be able to browse through books that may be of benefit and a list of hyperlinked online resources will be emailed out afterwards. We will verbally ask whether people would wish to be contacted again and whether they have suggestions for future workshops.

Workshop 3: community groups

This plan is adapted from work conducted within a community arts organisation, during a brief respite between Covid-19 lockdowns, with a pre-existing group of participants. Reference is made to outdoor spaces and recycled materials, but this was not always possible during tight restrictions.

Introduction: 15 minutes
Explain why we are here – to make a space to think about our relationship to nature and environment.

Quick introductions from each member of the group, including the facilitators

The aim of this activity is to raise awareness and appreciation of what is around us and what we carry around with us, using visual art to strengthen that connection. Make use of the 'In the Palm of Hand' quote if appropriate.

Explain that the objective is not about demonstrating individual acts of artistic skill, rather it is about exploring how we value what we have and noticing what we tend to overlook.

Individual activity: 30 minutes
Ask participants to consider one item they are carrying on them, whether on their person or in a bag, as a subject matter; if access to an outdoor space is possible, make use of this). Ideally, the item should fit into the palm of their hand.

Use only pencil or pens/paint to draw/paint what is in front of them. Keep the range of materials small. Participants can make multiple images if they wish.

Reflection: 15 minutes
Discussion of own work with the groups and feedback on activity.

Comfort break: 10 minutes

Individual activity: 30 minutes
Using reflections, ask participants to create a new piece of work, perhaps this could be with a different item or maybe using their imagination to illustrate their thoughts on the subject.

Participants are free to use colour as the choice of materials is wider, including the use of recycled materials and packaging. Participants can make multiple images if desired.

Reflection: 15 minutes
Discussion of own work with the group and feedback on activity. General discussion about theme of relationship to nature and the environment.

Close: 5 minutes
Thank people and provide written feedback forms.

Index